Hypertension
and Diabetes

3rd Edition

SCIENCE PRESS

Hypertension
and *Diabetes*

3rd Edition

AH Barnett BSc (Hons) MD FRCP
PM Dodson MDFRCP FRCOphth
Birmingham Heartlands Hospital
Birmingham, UK

With contributions by

Tahseen A Chowdhury MD ChB MRCP
Central Middlesex Hospital
London, UK

Mark J O'Donnell MB ChB MRCP
Blackpool Victoria Hospital
Blackpool, UK

SCIENCE PRESS

Published by Science Press Ltd, 34–42 Cleveland Street, London W1P 6LB, UK.

© 2000 Science Press Ltd.

http://current-science-group.com/

British Library Cataloguing in Publication Data.

A catalogue record for this book is available from the British Library.

ISBN 1-85873-902-0

Although every effort has been made to ensure that drug doses and other information are presented accurately in this publication, the ultimate responsibility rests with the prescribing physician. Neither the publishers nor the authors can be held responsible for errors or for any consequences arising from the use of information contained herein. Any product mentioned in this publication should be used in accordance with the prescribing information prepared by the manufacturers. No claims or endorsements are made for any drug or compound at present under clinical investigation.

Project editor: Clare Wheatcroft
Illustrator: Ian Potter
Designer: Simon Banister
Production: David Forrest

Printed in Italy by Programma

Cover illustration: Colour enhanced electron micrograph of a small blood vessel from a patient with long-standing diabetes.

Contents

Acknowledgements

Figure 1.3 Reprinted from Maxwell MH, Waks AU, Schroth PC *et al*. **Error in blood-pressure measurement due to incorrect cuff size in obese patients.** *Lancet* 1982, **2**:33–36, with permission from the BMJ Publishing Group.

Figure 1.4 Adapted with permission from Verdecchia P, Schillaci G, Guerrieri M *et al*. **Circadian blood pressure change and left ventricular hypertrophy in essential hypertension.** *Circulation* 1990, **81**:528–536.

Table 1.2 Reprinted from Turner RC, Millns H, Neil HA *et al*. **Risk factors for coronary artery disease in non-insulin dependent diabetes mellitus: United Kingdom Propective Diabetes Study (UKPDS 23).** *Br Med J* 1998, **316**:823–828, with permission from the BMJ Publishing Group.

Figure 2.5 Adapted with permission from Jennings PE, Barnett AH. **New approaches to the pathogenesis and treatment of diabetic microangiopathy.** *Diabet Med* 1988, **5**:111–117.

Figure 2.6 Adapted with permission from Giardino I, Brownlee M. **The biochemical basis of microvascular disease.** In *Textbook of Diabetes.* Second edition. Edited by JC Pickup and G Williams. Oxford: Blackwell Science Ltd, 1996.

Figure 3.4 Reprinted from Hostetter TH, Rennke HG, Brenner BM. **The case for intrarenal hypertension in the initiation and progression of diabetic and other glomerulopathies.** *Am J Med* 1982, **72**: 375–380, with permission from Excerpta Medica Inc.

Figure 3.5 Reprinted from Parving HH, Andersen AR, Smidt UM *et al*. **Early aggressive antihypertensive treatment reduces rate of decline in kidney function in diabetic nephropathy.** *Lancet* 1983, **1**: 1175–1179. © by The Lancet Ltd.

Figure 3.6 Adapted with permission from Davis JO. **What signals the kidney to release renin?** *Circ Res* 1971, **28**:301–306.

Figure 6.2 Reproduced with permission from PM Dodson, AH Barnett. *Lipids in Primary Care.* London: Medical Publishing Company, 1999.

Table 6.6 Reproduced with permission from Ramsay L, Williams B, Johnston G *et al*. **Guidelines for management of hypertension: report of the third working party of the British Hypertension Society.** *J Hum Hypertens* 1999, **13**:569–592.

Biographies

Anthony H Barnett BSc (Hons) MD FRCP qualified in Medicine at King's College Hospital, London, UK, in 1975, having previously obtained a first class honours degree in Pharmacology in 1972. He spent his early years in training at King's College Hospital, London, Walsgrave Hospital, Coventry and Leeds General Infirmary and then returned to the Diabetic Department at King's College Hospital in 1978 as a Clinical Registrar in Diabetic Medicine. This was followed by a post as Medical Research Council Senior Fellow at the same unit between 1979 and 1981. His MD thesis, entitled '*Aetiology of Diabetic Vascular Disease*', was followed by training as a Senior Registrar in Medicine, Diabetes and Endocrinology in New Zealand and Southampton. In 1983 he was appointed Senior Lecturer in Medicine and Diabetes and Honorary Consultant Physician at the University of Birmingham and Birmingham Heartlands Hospital. Subsequently, he was promoted to Reader in Medicine in 1989 and Professor of Medicine in 1992. His current research interests include the genetics of diabetes, susceptibility factors for microvascular complications and therapeutic interventions, with a particular interest in susceptibility factors for diabetic nephropathy, prevention and treatment.

Paul M Dodson MD FRCP FRCOphth qualified at St Bartholomew's Hospital, London, UK, in 1974. He spent his early years training at Southampton General Hospital and the Royal Berkshire Hospital in Reading. He returned to St Bartholomew's and Moorfields Eye Hospital, London, in 1979 to research diabetes, hyperlipidaemia and retinopathy, which led to his MD. He moved to Dudley Road Hospital (now City Hospital) in Birmingham as a Senior Registrar in Diabetes and Endocrinology, and completed studies on the nonpharmacological treatment and epidemiological aspects of hypertension in patients with diabetes. He was appointed Consultant Physician in Medicine, Diabetes and Endocrinology to Birmingham Heartlands Hospital and Honorary Senior Clinical Lecturer, University of Birmingham, in 1989. His current research interests include medical ophthamology (diabetic retinopathy and retinovascular disease), diabetes, hypertension and hyperlipidaemia.

Preface

Cardiovascular disease is now a major worldwide public health problem. It is set to overtake infectious diseases as the most common cause of death in many parts of the developing world, with the levels becoming comparable to those that have been seen in Western society for many years. The increasing prevalence of obesity, sedentary lifestyle and other lifestyle factors, including cigarette smoking, are all major contributors, and the co-occurrence of cardiovascular risk factors in the same person is now very commonly recognised. These cardiovascular risk factors include hypertension, diabetes, dyslipidaemia and cigarette smoking. The last few decades have seen an exponential rise in the prevalence of diabetes, particularly type 2 diabetes, all over the world, with estimates suggesting that 200 million people now suffer with the condition.

Although the major risk factors for cardiovascular disease are well recognised, evidence that improving these factors will reduce cardiovascular risk specifically in the population with diabetes has, until recently, been lacking. This has been a particular problem in the area of hypertension and diabetes since well over half of all people with diabetes have hypertension based on modern criteria! The last few years have, however, provided a major evidence base for the benefit of aggressive management of hypertension in patients with diabetes at a time when the latter has reached epidemic proportions in many parts of the world.

For the above reasons it gives us particular pleasure to edit the third edition of *Hypertension and Diabetes*. The first edition was published in 1990 and the second in 1996. Since then we have seen many published trials demonstrating the benefit of tight blood pressure control in patients with diabetes. These benefits include significant reductions in cardiovascular events and mortality. They have prompted the production of several new sets of guidelines for both thresholds for intervention and targets for treatment of blood pressure in these patients. The guidelines also emphasise that to achieve these targets the great majority of patients with diabetes will require at least two agents from different antihypertensive classes, and frequently more than two. Recent guidelines also emphasise the common co-occurrence of cardiovascular risk factors in the same patient including dyslipidaemia, cigarette smoking and obesity, and their active management. This has led to the concept of overall cardiovascular risk assessment in determining the need for pharmacotherapy.

Publication of these important trials, recommendations resulting from them for blood pressure control and emphasis on cardiovascular risk assessment, have all made it imperative that we produce a third edition of this book. We have added a chapter summarizing the various trials involving diabetic patients with hypertension and have re-written other chapters to take into account more recent information. Recent trials in this area have mainly focused on cardiovascular disease, but we have also covered the important and convincing evidence that hypertension is a major risk factor for progression of small vessel disease (retinopathy and nephropathy), and the evidence that tight control of blood pressure is of benefit.

We have tried to produce a readable and practical update that will be of interest and help to all professionals working in this important area. We hope we have succeeded!

AH Barnett
PM Dodson

Epidemiology and pathogenesis of hypertension in diabetes

Macrovascular disease is the major cause of morbidity and mortality in people with diabetes in the UK, the USA and many other countries [1]. Attempts to improve prognosis must address this central observation. Hypertension is recognised as a major risk factor for cardiovascular disease (Figure 1.1) and cerebrovascular disease (Figure 1.2). This chapter is concerned with the epidemiology and pathogenesis of hypertension in diabetes. Although the discussion is principally of hypertension, other risk factors including smoking, hypercholesterolaemia, obesity and hyperglycaemia are also considered.

Post-mortem specimen of a large cerebral infarction with haemorrhage in the left cerebral hemisphere

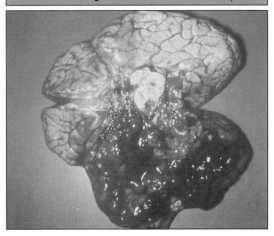

Figure 1.2

Post-mortem specimen of myocardial infarction in the left ventricle

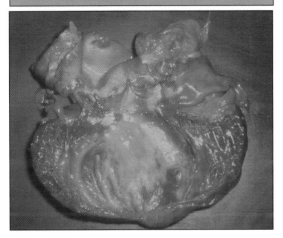

Figure 1.1

Definition of hypertension in patients with diabetes

Over the last few years, extensive randomized trial data have led to a revision of the definition of hypertension by a number of national and international bodies. The World Health Organization (WHO) and International Society of Hypertension (ISH) [2] state in their 1999 guidelines that hypertension is defined as a systolic blood pressure of 140 mmHg or greater and/or a diastolic blood pressure of 90 mmHg or greater, in patients who are not taking antihypertensive medication. The blood pressure values for patients with diabetes are generally agreed by the guidelines of the USA Joint National Committee (JNC), the JNC-VI [3]; by the guidelines of the British Hypertension Society (BHS) [4]; and the joint British societies' guidelines [5]. The guidelines place emphasis not only on blood pressure, but also on the presence of other cardiovascular risk factors and hence overall cardiovascular risk. While there has been debate on the relative importance of systolic and diastolic blood pressure, in practice systolic blood pressure should be regarded as the more important.

Blood pressure measurement

Blood pressure must be accurately and correctly measured, using a Cuscoe's cuff and taken after five minutes rest. There should be a correction for obesity by using a wider sphygmomanometer cuff if the mid-arm circumference is greater than 33 cm [6]. A standard blood pressure cuff has been shown to overestimate blood pressure in obese patients (Figure 1.3) [6]. Blood pressure should be measured

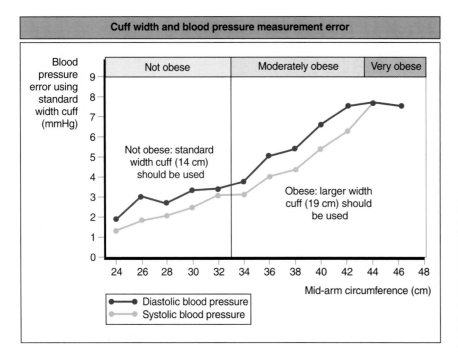

Cuff width and blood pressure measurement error

Blood pressure error using standard width cuff (mmHg)

Not obese | Moderately obese | Very obese

Not obese: standard width cuff (14 cm) should be used

Obese: larger width cuff (19 cm) should be used

Mid-arm circumference (cm)

● Diastolic blood pressure
● Systolic blood pressure

Figure 1.3. Using a standard sphygmo-manometer cuff when measuring the blood pressure of obese patients increases the margin of error of measurement. This illustrates the importance of measuring the mid-arm circumference. Reproduced with permission from [6].

in the supine or sitting position, particularly if there is evidence of autonomic dysfunction. Since the medical use of mercury is likely to be restricted around the world, the calibration and accuracy of non-mercury devices will become increasingly important.

Although the blood pressure levels quoted in prevalence and treatment trials of hypertension are based on one casual reading, this is clinically insufficient to determine the diagnosis of hyper-tension; repeated measurements generally pro-duce reduced average blood pressure estimates. A diagnosis of hypertension should be made on the basis of three or more separate blood pressure examinations (*see* Chapter 6).

Non-invasive ambulatory blood pressure monitoring (ABPM) has advanced significantly over recent years with devices that are quiet in operation, weigh less than a kilogram and will record blood pressure without the measurement itself producing a pressor effect [7]. ABPM removes many of the inaccuracies of blood pressure measurement in the clinic with the standard sphygmomanometer. In particular, elimination of observer bias, identification of 'white coat' hypertension and assessment of blood pres-sure control may be made with ABPM (Table 1.1).

A considerable advantage of ABPM is its repro-ducibility: it usually averages over 20 measure-

Clinical situations in which ambulatory blood pressure monitoring may be indicated

- When blood pressure shows unusual variability
- To diagnose 'white coat' hypertension (elevated clinic reading, normal ambulatory blood pressure monitoring)
- In hypertension resistant to drug therapy (>150/90 mmHg), on a regimen of three of more antihypertensive drugs
- When symptoms suggest the possibility of hypotension

Table 1.1

ments to obtain the blood pressure status for an individual [8].

An example of blood pressure patterns throughout a 24-hour period in normal and hypertensive patients is shown in Figure 1.4 [9]. In the normotensive indi-vidual, blood pressures are lower at night, with a decline in systolic and diastolic blood pressure of more than 10/5 mmHg compared with daytime mea-surements (the nocturnal dip). In people with essen-tial hypertension, blood pressure is elevated and sustained during the day with less nocturnal dip (referred to as non-dipping). Blood pressure mea-surements taken by ABPM have also been shown to

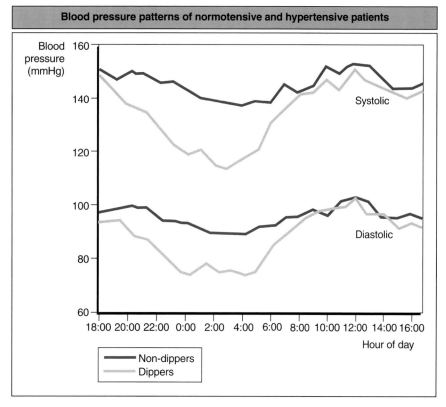

Blood pressure patterns of normotensive and hypertensive patients

Systolic

Diastolic

Non-dippers
Dippers

Hour of day

Figure 1.4. The blood pressure was recorded by ambulatory blood pressure monitoring. Those patients who have a nocturnal dip in blood pressure of less than 10% of their daytime value are termed 'non-dippers'. Adapted with permission from [9].

relate more closely to a range of target organ damage (TOD) in individuals with hypertension than clinical blood pressure measurements [10]. These TODs include left ventricular hypertrophy (LVH), microalbuminuria, lacunar cerebral infarctions and retinal vessel abnormalities. LVH is one of the most powerful predictors of cardiovascular disease and the closer relationship of ABPM measurements to LVH is a clear advantage for the technique. ABPM is becoming more widely used in patients with diabetes to confirm or refute the diagnosis of hypertension and is playing a more prominent role in antihypertensive management [11]. An example of its use is shown in Table 1.2 [12].

Prevalence of hypertension in diabetes

Hypertension occurs more commonly among people with type 1 and type 2 diabetes than in the general population. The early clinical studies suggested a strong relationship between hypertension and diabetes [13] but, because of the numerous problems of methodology, many of these papers were difficult

to interpret [14]. Subsequent reduction of the levels of blood pressure defining hypertension meant that the existing estimates of prevalence were shown to be significantly underestimated.

Most studies using the revised criteria for hypertension (previously defined as 160/90–95 mmHg or lower), including large population studies (Framingham study, Whitehall and Bedford study and UK Prospective Diabetes study [UKPDS] [12,15,16]), confirm the higher rate of prevalence. These studies demonstrate prevalence rates for hypertension in diabetes of 32% in men and 45% in women (Table 1.2) [12]. These figures are similar to clinical practice; in a district general hospital diabetic clinic, for example, 40% (203/507) of patients with diabetes under the age of 65 years had hypertension according to the earlier WHO criteria (Figure 1.5) [17,18]. Interestingly, there appeared to be differences between the ethnic groups. People of West Indian origin with diabetes had a greater prevalence (49%) of hypertension than subjects of either white (37%) or Asian (35%) origin. There was a higher incidence of hyperten-

Principal findings of UKPDS cardiovascular risk factor studyin type 2 diabetes (1998)		
	Men (_n_=1,564)	**Women (_n_=1,129)**
Mean age (years)	52	53
Body mass index (kg/m²)	27.1	29.4
Systolic blood pressure (mmHg)	133±18	139±20
Diastolic blood pressure (mmHg)	82±10	83±10
Patients with hypertension (%)	32	45
Current smokers (%)	32	29
Stepwise selection of risk factors for coronary artery disease*		
1) Low-density lipoprotein cholesterol		
2) High-density lipoprotein cholesterol (negative)		
3) Haemoglobin A1c		
4) Systolic blood pressure		
5) Smoking		

Table 1.2. UKPDS, UK Prospective Diabetes Study; *median duration of follow-up 7.8 years. Reproduced with permission from [12].

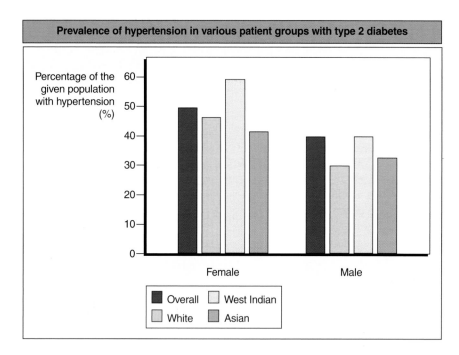

Figure 1.5. The results are from a district hospital diabetic clinic. Data from [17,18].

sion in women than in men, a trend confirmed in other studies. This study [17] also emphasised the common occurrence of isolated systolic hypertension in patients with type 2 diabetes (Table 1.3) [17,18]. Malignant or accelerated hypertension is recorded as rare in people with diabetes, but the authors suspect this is more common than has been previously appreciated because of the incor-

rect classification of hypertensive retinal changes as diabetic retinopathy.

There may be distinct geographical variation in the frequency of hypertension in diabetes. The WHO multinational study of vascular disease and diabetes included 6,695 men and women with diabetes between the ages of 35 and 54 years from 14 centres throughout Europe [19]. The overall propor-

Types of hypertension in patients with type 2 diabetes		
	Men (%)	Women (%)
Isolated systolic hypertension	48	60
Isolated diastolic hypertension	5	2
Systolic and diastolic hypertension	32	19
Normotensive with therapy	13.5	19

Table 1.3. Data from [17,18].

tion of patients with diabetes and hypertension was 36%, but within the European capital cities values ranged from 22% in London to 38% in Berlin.

Prevalence rates from other centres, including ones in the USA and Asia, showed values ranging from 26% to 36%. Africa was not included here, but another study from Nigeria compared 402 patients with diabetes with a matched control group and showed an increased prevalence of hypertension in the group with diabetes (37% versus 27%) [20].

Some studies have investigated the blood pressure differences between patients with type 1 and type 2 diabetes. A significantly higher prevalence of hypertension is associated with type 1 diabetes, but this probably relates to the presence of diabetic nephropathy, as the prevalence of hypertension and diabetic nephropathy in this population is similar [21].

Sound evidence exists for an increased frequency of hypertension in patients with type 1 and type 2 diabetes. All the data have been analysed using the earlier, higher levels of blood pressure as the definition of hypertension, and therefore the true prevalence of hypertension is likely to be nearer 70%, using the most recent definition of hypertension of 140/90 mmHg or greater. In the elderly, hypertension is predominately systolic; in younger patients the relationship with diastolic hypertension is less clear. This latter finding may reflect the difference in aetiology of hypertension in the two age groups. There is firm evidence that hypertension associated with type 1 diabetes relates to the presence of incipient or overt diabetic nephropathy [22,23] (*see* Chapter 3).

Aetiology of hypertension associated with diabetes

The aetiology of hypertension in association with diabetes, as with that of essential hypertension, is incompletely understood and is complicated by the fact that pathogenesis may differ between the two types of diabetes. Hypertension in type 1 diabetes is related to the development of diabetic nephropathy, which is not usually the case in type 2 diabetes [21–24]. A list of possible pathways is shown in Table 1.4 and a schematic representation of their interaction in Figure 1.6.

The chronic cardiovascular risk factor syndrome (syndrome X)

In 1988, Gerald Reaven proposed that the term 'syndrome X' should be applied to a series of related variables that are important in the genesis of coronary artery disease [25]. These include insulin resistance, hyperinsulinaemia, abnormal glucose tolerance, lipid abnormalities and hypertension (Table 1.5).

This proposal arose from a number of clinical observations [26–28]. In non-obese individuals with essential hypertension, the non-oxidative pathway of insulin-mediated glucose disposal is impaired; the site of this disturbance is predominantly skeletal muscle. Resistance to insulin-stimulated glucose uptake is a common phenomenon and a characteristic finding in patients with type 2 diabetes and impaired glucose tolerance. If an individual is overweight, particularly if there is central obesity,

Major factors possibly involved in the pathogenesis of hypertension associated with **diabetes**
• Obesity
• Nephropathy
• Hyperinsulinaemia
• Sodium retention
• Catecholamines
• Renin–angiotensin system
• Atrial natriuretic peptide
• Renal artery stenosis
• Arteriosclerosis
• Leptin

Table 1.4

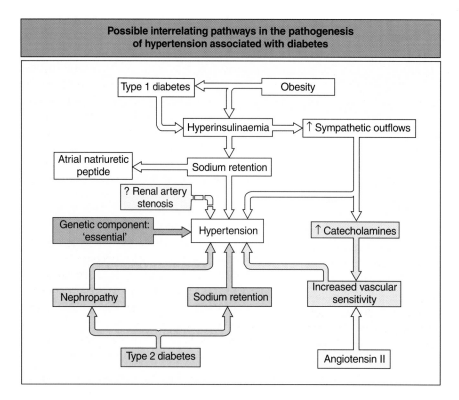

Possible interrelating pathways in the pathogenesis of hypertension associated with diabetes

Figure 1.6

Suggested component features of syndrome X
• Insulin resistance
• Hyperinsulinaemia
• Glucose intolerance
• Increased very-low-density lipoprotein
• Decreased high-density lipoprotein
• Hypertension

Table 1.5

insulin resistance is a common feature [26]. Furthermore, insulin resistance is more marked in obese individuals who have hypertension than in those who are normotensive.

The effects of hyperinsulinaemia and insulin resistance, will impact on other systems, which may relate to the presence of hypertension. For example, insulin is known to stimulate the sympathetic nervous system, resulting in a significant elevation in plasma catecholamine concentrations [29]. The sodium-retaining properties of insulin, probably acting at the level of the proximal tubule, are also well-documented [30]. This

should increase total exchangeable body sodium as well as total vascular volume, and in type 2 diabetes increased total body sodium is a consistent finding [24]. Lipoprotein lipase, which is the major clearance enzyme of triglyceride-rich particles in the periphery, is insulin sensitive [31]. In the presence of insulin resistance, low high-density lipoprotein (HDL) cholesterol and increased very-low-density lipoprotein (VLDL) concentrations are a major feature.

Whether either or both of insulin resistance and hyperinsulinaemia promote the development of hypertension is unclear. Acute hyperinsulinaemia produces vasodilatation [32], sympathetic activation [29], enhanced renal sodium absorption [30], and possible chronotropic and inotropic effects [33]. Systemic arterial blood pressure is increased when insulin is given in physiological doses, but falls when the sympathetic response is insufficient and with chronic administration of insulin. Hyperinsulinaemia might, however, increase vascular resistance and blood pressure through stimulation of vascular smooth muscle cell proliferation [34] or alternatively through vasoconstriction caused by an as yet unidentified insulin resistance at the vascular level [35].

A genetic predisposition is a likely link between hypertension and diabetes. Recent studies have shown that a family history of hypertension is more common among relatives of patients with type 2 diabetes than type 1 diabetes. Reports have found an increased prevalence of parental hypertension for young men with type 2 diabetes and high blood pressure [36,37]. This suggests that part of the hypertension associated with diabetes may be of the familial, essential type. This aspect was also studied in 91 patients with type 1 diabetes and 183 with type 2 diabetes [38]. Allowing for age and body mass index, the risk of hypertension in siblings of these patients was found to be greater in those with a diabetic parent with hypertension compared with those with a normotensive parent. The implication from this study is that there is a link between hypertension and diabetes and that it is of the 'essential' form. In patients with type 1 diabetes, a genetic predisposition for hypertension has been suggested, by the finding of altered sodium–lithium countertransport in erythrocytes, as a risk factor for the development of diabetic nephropathy [39]; this also facilitates the rise in blood pressure that tends to occur before or with the development of nephropathy [39]. Disappointingly, studies of the various angiotensin-converting enzyme (ACE) genotypes in hypertension and coronary artery disease have not shown a clear link [40].

Other factors

Abnormalities in a number of systems may be relevant in the hypertension associated with diabetes. Activation of the renin–angiotensin system (RAS) causes a pressor response mediated by angiotensin II combined with aldosterone-induced sodium retention. In uncomplicated diabetes, plasma renin activity has been reported as high, normal, or low [41–43]. An increased vascular sensitivity to angiotensin II has been observed in patients with diabetes, and improvement of metabolic control normalizes circulating angiotensin II and aldosterone levels [44].

Although basal levels of plasma catecholamines (both noradrenaline and adrenaline) are normal in patients with diabetes compared with age-matched control subjects [41], evidence shows that in diabetes there may be an altered vascular sensitivity to catecholamines [45]. This altered vascular sensitivity appears to be independent of age, duration of diabetes, or type of therapy.

Neural pathway defects have been studied, as impaired glucose tolerance and hypertension may represent a common pathophysiological pathway. Major neuronally mediated mechanisms in hypertension may be a direct primary increase or baroreceptor-mediated increase in sympathetic output, which may be important in diabetes as an increase in sympathetic activity has been shown to be a direct effect of insulin [29]. The principle neuro-endocrine pathways that may provide a common link are the endogenous opiate system and the central RAS.

Diabetic nephropathy

Hypertension in type 1 diabetes relates to diabetic nephropathy. The situation has become clear with studies of the early markers of diabetic renal disease, particularly microalbuminuria (*see* Chapter 3). Reports have shown that patients with diabetes and microalbuminuria have significantly higher blood pressure values than matched patients with diabetes and normal protein excretion [45,46].

Renal histopathological studies in diabetic patients with hypertension are of interest [47]. In a sample of 250 renal biopsy specimens from patients with diabetes and hypertension, there was a high incidence of arteriosclerosis, glomerulosclerosis and pyelonephritis; 93% of patients with hypertension had arteriosclerosis and there was a strong correlation between the extent of the lesion and the level of blood pressure. Some patients were, however, found to have glomerulonephritis, particularly of the membranous type. This supports the suggestion that hypertension in patients with diabetes and renal involvement may be the result of renal lesions other than those of 'classic' or typical diabetic nephropathy.

An area of practical concern is renal artery stenosis. Diabetes is associated with accelerated atherosclerosis and it is likely that some patients with diabetes have a degree of atheromatous renal artery stenosis [48]. Although this may contribute to hypertension in the patient with diabetes, its precise prevalence in patients with diabetes with or without hypertension is not clear and may, in part, be a reflection of physicians' unwillingness to perform renal angiograms. In a retrospective study of autopsy data, a 3.5-fold increase in renal artery stenosis in patients with diabetes was observed, but a limited number of clinical studies have questioned whether the stenoses were

Endocrine causes of diabetes and hypertension
• Thyrotoxicosis
• Phaeochromocytoma
• Cushing's syndrome
• Acromegaly
• Synthetic oestrogen and progesterone combination therapy

Table 1.6

haemodynamically significant [49]. The use of ACE inhibitors in current therapy makes the further study of this important because of the potential deterioration in renal function with this class of drugs in patients with renal artery stenosis.

Endocrine causes

Some patients develop hypertension and diabetes secondary to another endocrine cause (Table 1.6). Although it is extremely important to identify these cases, as effective treatment may be available, the conditions (with the exception of thyrotoxicosis) are rare.

Multiple risk factors

Hypertension and diabetes can no longer be viewed in isolation as risk factors for coronary and cardiovascular disease. The frequent co-occurrence of cardiovascular risk factors (components of syndrome X and smoking), in addition to the additive effect on coronary risk, have heralded a change in approach and management. Data from the UKPDS study arms (Table 1.2) and others demonstrate the devastating results of diabetes on cardiovascular and microvascular disease outcome, emphasising that focus on overall cardiovascular risk is necessary (*see* Chapters 5 and 6).

Summary

An association between hypertension and diabetes is clearly established, with up to 70% of patients with diabetes having hypertension. Although the exact pathogenesis is unclear, it is likely that the aetiological mechanisms of hypertension between the two types of diabetes are different. Diabetic nephropathy may account for the increased prevalence of hypertension in patients with type 1 diabetes and hyperinsulinaemia (or insulin resistance) may contribute in patients with type 2 diabetes.

References

1. Panzram G. **Mortality and survival in type II (non-insulin-dependent) diabetes mellitus.** *Diabetologia* 1987, **30**:123–131.

2. Anonymous. **1999 World Health Organisation–International Society of Hypertension Guidelines for the Management of Hypertension. Guidelines Subcommittee.** *J Hypertens* 1999, **17**:151–183.

3. Anonymous. **The sixth report of the Joint National Committee on prevention, detection, evaluation, and treatment of high blood pressure.** *Arch Intern Med* 1997, **157**:2413–2446.

4. Ramsay L, Williams B, Johnston G *et al.* **Guidelines for management of hypertension: report of the third working party of the British Hypertension Society.** *J Hum Hypertens* 1999, **13**:569–592.

5. Anonymous. **Joint British recommendations on prevention of coronary heart disease in clinical practice.** *Heart* 1998, **80** (suppl. 2):S1–S29.

6. Maxwell MH, Waks AU, Schroth PC *et al.* **Error in blood-pressure measurement due to incorrect cuff size in obese patients.** *Lancet* 1982, **2**:33–36.

7. Parati G, Pomidossi G, Casadei R *et al.* **Lack of altering reactions to intermittent cuff inflations during non-invasive pressure monitoring.** *Hypertension* 1985, **7**:597–601.

8. Conway J, Johnston J, Coats A *et al.* **The use of ambulatory blood pressure monitoring to improve the accuracy and reduce the numbers of subjects in clinical trials of antihypertensive agents.** *J Hypertens* 1988, **6**:111–116.

9. Verdecchia P, Schillaci G, Guerrieri M *et al.* **Circadian blood pressure change and left ventricular hypertrophy in essential hypertension.** *Circulation* 1990, **81**:528–536.

10. Staessen JA, Thijs L, Fagard R *et al.* **Predicting cardiovascular risk using conventional vs ambulatory blood pressure in older patients with systolic hypertension. Systolic Hypertension in Europe Trial Investigators.** *JAMA* 1999, **282**:539–546.

11. Stanton AV. **Prediction of cardiovascular damage in hypertensive patients: clinic or ambulatory blood pressures?** *J Hum Hypertens* 1999, **13**:81–83.

12. Turner RC, Millns H, Neil HA *et al.* **Risk factors for coronary artery disease in non-insulin dependent diabetes mellitus: United Kingdom Prospective Diabetes Study.** *Br Med J* 1998, **316**:823–828.

13. Drury PL. **Diabetes and arterial hypertension.** *Diabetologia* 1983, **24**:1–9.

14. Pacy PJ. **Hypertension and diabetes mellitus.** In *Diabetes and the Heart.* Edited by KG Taylor. Tunbridge Wells, Kent: Castle House Publications, 1987;42–60.

15. Kannel WB, McGee DL. **Diabetes and cardiovascular disease. The Framingham study.** *JAMA* 1979, **241**:2035–2038.

16. Jarrett RJ, Keen H, McCartney M *et al.* **Glucose tolerance and blood pressure in two population samples:**

their relation to diabetes mellitus and hypertension. *Int J Epidemiol* 1978, **7**:15–24.

17. Pacy PJ, Dodson PM, Beevers M *et al.* **Prevalence of hypertension in white, black and Asian diabetics in a district hospital diabetic clinic.** *Diabetic Med* 1985, **2**:125–130.

18. Barret-Connor E, Criqui MH, Klauber MR *et al.* **Diabetes and hypertension in a community of older adults.** *Am J Epidemiol* 1981, **113**:276–284.

19. World Health Organisation. *Vascular Disease in Diabetics. Report of WHO Multinational Study of Vascular Disease in Diabetes.* Geneva: WHO 1982;1–93.

20. Oli JM, Ikeh VO. **Diabetes mellitus and hypertension in an African population.** *J R Coll Physicians Lond* 1986, **20**:32–35.

21. Christlieb AR, Warram JH, Krolewaki AS *et al.* **Hypertension: the major risk factor in juvenile-onset insulin-dependent diabetics.** *Diabetes* 1981, **30** (suppl. 2):90–96.

22. Parving HH, Hommel E. **Prognosis in diabetic nephropathy.** *Br Med J* 1989, **299**:230–233.

23. Borch-Johnsen K, Andersen PK, Deckert T. **The effect of proteinuria on relative mortality in type I (insulin-dependent) diabetes mellitus.** *Diabetologia* 1985, **28**:590–596.

24. Dodson PM, Horton RC. **The hypertension of diabetes mellitus: mechanisms and implications.** *J Hum Hypertens* 1988, **1**:241–247.

25. Reaven GM. **Banting lecture 1988. Role of insulin resistance in human disease.** *Diabetes* 1988, **37**:1595–1607.

26. Modan M, Halkin H, Almog S *et al.* **Hyperinsulinaemia. A link between hypertension, obesity and glucose intolerance.** *J Clin Invest* 1985, **75**:809–817.

27. Bain SC, Dodson PM. **The chronic cardiovascular risk factor syndrome (syndrome X): mechanisms and implications for atherogenesis.** *Postgrad Med J* 1991, **67**:922–927.

28. Landin K, Krotkiewski M, Smith U. **Importance of obesity for the metabolic abnormalities associated with an abdominal fat distribution.** *Metabolism* 1989, **38**:572–576.

29. Rowe JW, Young JB, Minaker KL *et al.* **Effect of insulin and glucose infusions on sympathetic nervous system activity in normal man.** *Diabetes* 1981, **30**:219–225.

30. DeFronzo RA. **The effect of insulin on renal sodium metabolism. A review with clinical implications.** *Diabetologia* 1981, **21**:165–171.

31. Bain SC. **The effects of diabetes on lipoprotein metabolism.** In *Lipid, Diabetes and Vascular Disease. Second edition.* Edited by PM Dodson and AH Barnett. London: Science Press, 1998;15–23.

32. Anderson EA, Mark AL. **The vasodilator action of insulin. Implications for the insulin hypothesis of hypertension.** *Hypertension* 1993, **21**:136–141.

33. Ferrari P, Weidmann P. **Insulin, insulin sensitivity and hypertension.** *Hypertension* 1990, **8**:491–500.

34. Stout RW. **Insulin as a mitogenic factor: role in the pathogenesis of cardiovascular disease.** *Am J Med* 1991, **90** (suppl. 2A):62S–65S.

35. Ferriss JB. **The causes of raised blood pressure in insulin dependent and non-insulin dependent diabetes.** *J Hum Hypertens* 1991, **5**:245–254.

36. Krolewski AS, Czyzyk A, Kopazynski J *et al.* **Prevalence of diabetes mellitus, coronary heart disease and hypertension in the families of insulin dependent and insulin independent diabetes.** *Diabetologia* 1987, **21**:520–524.

37. Tarn AC, Drury PL. **Blood pressure in children, adolescents and young adults with type I (insulin-dependent) diabetes.** *Diabetologia* 1986, **29**:275–281.

38. Kelleher C, Kingston SM, Barry DG *et al.* **Hypertension in diabetic clinic patients and their siblings.** *Diabetologia* 1988, **31**:76–81.

39. Viberti GC, Earle K. **Predisposition to essential hypertension and the development of diabetic nephropathy.** *J Am Soc Nephrol* 1992, **3** (suppl.):S27–S33.

40. Jeunemaitre X, Lifton RP, Hunt SC *et al.* **Absence of linkage between the angiotensin converting enzyme locus and human essential hypertension.** *Nat Genet* 1992, **1**:72–75.

41. de Châtel R, Weidmann P, Flammer J *et al.* **Sodium, renin, aldosterone, catecholamines, and blood pressure in diabetes mellitus.** *Kidney Int* 1977, **12**:412–421.

42. Anderson S, Jung FF, Ingelfinger JR. **Renal renin–angiotensin system in diabetes: functional, immunohistochemical, and molecular biological correlations.** *Am J Physiol* 1993, **265**:F477–F486.

43. Beretta-Piccoli C, Weidmann P, Keusch G. **Responsiveness of plasma renin and aldosterone in diabetes mellitus.** *Kidney Int* 1981, **20**:259–266.

44. O'Hare JA, Ferriss JB, Twomey BM *et al.* **Changes in blood pressure, body fluids, circulating angiotensin II and aldosterone with improved diabetic control.** *Clin Sci* 1982, **63**:415S–418S.

45. Winocour PH, Durrington PN, Ishola M *et al.* **Influence of proteinuria on vascular disease, blood pressure, and lipoprotein in insulin dependent diabetes mellitus.** *Br Med J (Clin Res Ed)* 1987, **294**:1648–1651.

46. Wiegmann TB, Herron KG, Chonko AM *et al.* **Recognition of hypertension and abnormal blood pressure burden with ambulatory blood pressure recordings in type I diabetes mellitus.** *Diabetes* 1990, **39**:1556–1560.

47. Ditscherlein G. **Renal histopathology in hypertensive diabetic patients.** *Hypertension* 1984, **7** (suppl. II):29–32.

48. Sawicki PT, Kaiser S, Heinemann L *et al.* **Prevalence of renal artery stenosis in diabetes mellitus – an autopsy study.** *J Intern Med* 1991, **229**:489–492.

49. Wachtell K, Ibsen H, Olsen MH *et al.* **Prevalence of renal artery stenosis in patients with peripheral vascular disease and hypertension.** *J Hum Hypertens* 1996, **10**:83–85.

Hypertension as a risk factor for diabetic vascular disease

Hypertension is approximately twice as common in the population with diabetes compared with the population without diabetes [1,2] (*see* Chapter 1). There is increasing evidence that hypertension associated with diabetes is a risk factor for both large and small vessel disease.

Large vessel disease (macrovascular disease)

The major risk factors [3–6] are:

- hypertension;
- dyslipidaemia;
- diabetes;
- cigarette smoking; and
- positive family history.

These risk factors commonly co-occur in the same patient and this is particularly relevant to those with type 2 diabetes. Large vessel disease is by far the greatest cause of morbidity and premature death in patients with diabetes [3,4,7–11]. In particular, atherosclerotic disease that involves the coronary, cerebral and peripheral vessels occurs at an earlier age and with greater frequency in patients with diabetes, although the pathological features appear the same as in patients without diabetes.

The essential lesion is in accelerated atherosclerosis, and alterations in endothelial cell and platelet interactions, and in lipid and lipoprotein metabolism have all been implicated. Hyperglycaemia and increased levels of low-density lipoprotein (LDL) and VLDL may adversely affect vascular endothelium [12]. Hypertension increases the risk of vascular endothelial injury with subsequent macrophage and platelet aggregation, the release of growth factors that stimulate the proliferation of smooth muscle cells and the deposition of lipid-laden foam cells.

Coronary heart disease

Patients with diabetes, particularly women, have twice the risk of coronary heart disease (CHD). The generally higher mortality rate from CHD in patients with diabetes may be explained by the increased interplay of multiple risk factors (*see* Chapter 1), although diabetes *per se* is also an independent risk factor [13].

Cerebrovascular disease

Both hypertension and diabetes significantly increase the risk of cerebrovascular accident, and transient ischaemic episodes have been reported to occur between two and six times more frequently in people with diabetes [14–17]. Cerebrovascular accident occurs twice as often in diabetic patients with hypertension as in those with hypertension alone [16–18].

Peripheral vascular disease

A patient with diabetes over the age of 70 years has a 70-fold increased risk of peripheral gangrene compared with a subject without diabetes of the same age. Presentation may include symptoms of intermittent claudication, rest pain, arterial foot ulceration (Figure 2.1), peripheral gangrene (Figure 2.2) and infection. In the older patient with diabetes in particular, there appears to be a close correlation between systolic hypertension and peripheral vascular disease [19,20]. It is not clear, however, whether hypertension causes the vascular disease or merely reflects the altered physical properties of the vessels [21].

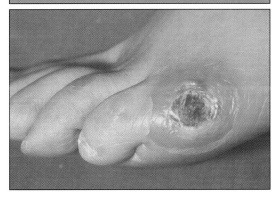

Typical arterial (ischaemic) ulcer at base of the small toe

Figure 2.1. The centre of this arterial ulcer is necrotic, with little callous formation. These ulcers are often painful.

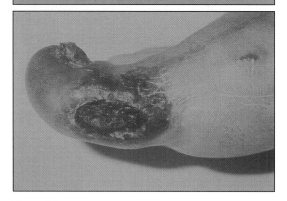

Figure 2.2

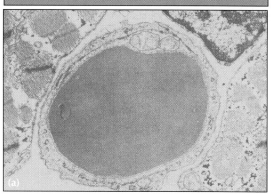

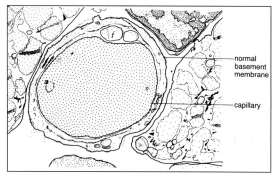

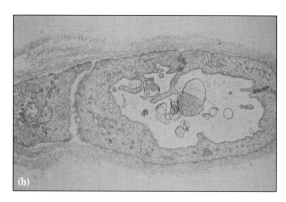

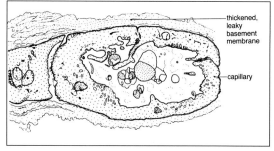

Small vessel disease (microangiopathy)

This disorder of the small blood vessels (Figure 2.3), specific to diabetes, is clinically apparent in the eyes (retinopathy), kidneys (nephropathy), vasa nervorum of peripheral nerves (neuropathy), and perhaps the myocardium of the heart (cardiomyopathy). Retinopathy is still the commonest cause of blindness in the working population of the developed world, and nephropathy is the cause of death in 20–35% of patients with type 1 diabetes [7–9] and of an unknown, but significant, proportion of patients with type 2 diabetes. Hypertension might be an initiating factor in the pathogenesis of these disorders and is certainly a major risk factor for progression.

Pathogenesis of microangiopathy

The major susceptibility factors for microangiopathy are duration of disease and metabolic control [22–24], while the actual development probably reflects many factors including:

- functional abnormalities within the microcirculation [25];
- pathophysiological consequences of enhanced glucose metabolism by different pathways of non-glycolytic metabolism [26]; and
- hypertension.

Specific processes involved include non-enzymatic glycosylation and formation of advanced glycosylation end products from long-lived tissue proteins (Figure 2.4) [26,27]. During this process glucose

Figure 2.3. (a) The small blood vessel of a non-diabetic person shows normal basement membrane appearances. **(b)** The basement membrane of a patient with long-standing diabetes is abnormal and thickened and will tend to leak plasma protein.

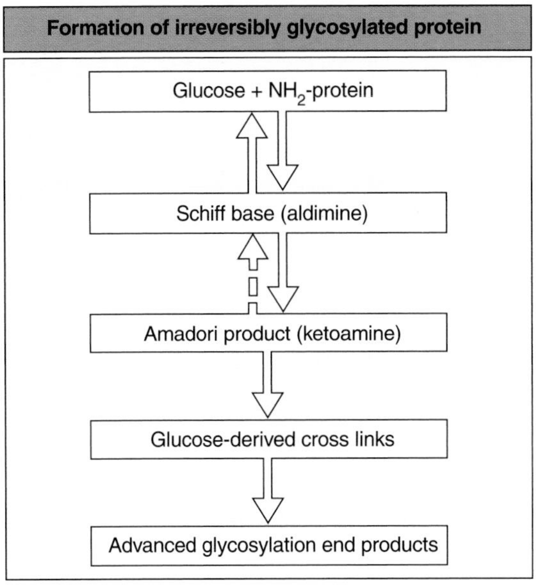

Formation of irreversibly glycosylated protein

Glucose + NH$_2$-protein

⇅

Schiff base (aldimine)

⇅

Amadori product (ketoamine)

⇩

Glucose-derived cross links

⇩

Advanced glycosylation end products

Figure 2.4. Non-enzymatic glycosylation produces first a Schiff base (freely reversible). In the presence of continuing hyperglycaemia, this is followed by ketoamine formation (partially reversible) and, finally, advanced glycosylation end products (irreversible). These products accumulate indefinitely in long-lived tissue proteins, for example, collagen, causing capillary basement membrane damage.

attaches to long-lived tissue proteins such as collagen to form a Schiff base (a non-enzymatic reaction). This reaction is reversible, but in the presence of continuing hyperglycaemia an Amadori product (ketoamine) is produced. Even at this stage the process may be slowly and partially reversible, but a continuing high glucose level results in the formation of advanced glycoslation end products, which continue to accumulate indefinitely on long-lived proteins because the reaction involved in their formation is irreversible. This process may be responsible for the excessive accumulation of basement membrane collagen seen in microangiopathy. In addition, these proteins trap potentially damaging immunoglobulin and complement components, thus contributing to a vicious circle of vascular damage. Hyperglycaemia also stimulates the intracellular polyol pathway [28,29].

Aldose reductase activity has been demonstrated in all tissues involved in the microangiopathic process. Sorbitol dehydrogenase is the rate-limiting step resulting in sorbitol accumulation. Reduced nicotinamide adenine dinucleotide phosphate (NADPH) is an important cofactor in the intracellular conversion of glucose to sorbitol. Excessive production of NADPH results in defective redox cycling and lower levels of reduced antioxidants, which are required to scavenge free radicals. Free radicals are violently reactive chemical species, produced during the course of normal metabolism, which contain an unpaired electron in their structure. They are thus powerful oxidants, causing lipid peroxidation and protein denaturation and aggregation. The consequences of these metabolic processes include capillary endothelial cell damage and dysfunction, and increased platelet aggregation, contributing to a vicious circle involving release of factors such as platelet factor 4, thromboxane and factor VIII [26].

The above is associated with various haemostatic abnormalities including increased fibrinogen, and decreased fibrinolysis. This results in an imbalance between thromboxane (vasoconstricting and platelet aggregating) and prostacyclin (vasodilating and anti-aggregating) in favour of thromboxane [26].

The sequence above culminates in capillary basement membrane abnormalities (Figure 2.3), protein leakage, microthrombus formation and tissue ischaemia. These factors, together with haemodynamic abnormalities such as hypertension, genetic susceptibility and perhaps insulin-like growth factors [30], result in the microvascular changes seen in susceptible target organs (Figure 2.5) [26].

Data largely accruing within the last decade have also suggested a role for diacyl glycerol synthesis and increased protein kinase C (PKC) activation in the development of diabetic microvascular disease (Figure 2.6) [28,31,32]. Hyperglycaemia is associated with increased glucose flux across membranes and increased synthesis of diacyl glycerol, which in turn activates PKC. Increased PKC activity is associated with increased vascular permeability, blood flow changes, basement membrane synthesis and stimulation of growth factors such as vascular endothelial growth factor. This pathway may relate to some of the more traditional pathways described above and in particular may be linked to intracellular glycation.

Trials are underway to study the effects of PKC inhibitors in diabetic retinopathy, nephropathy, neuropathy and erectile dysfunction [31].

Hypertension influences the various clinically important complications associated with microangiopathy.

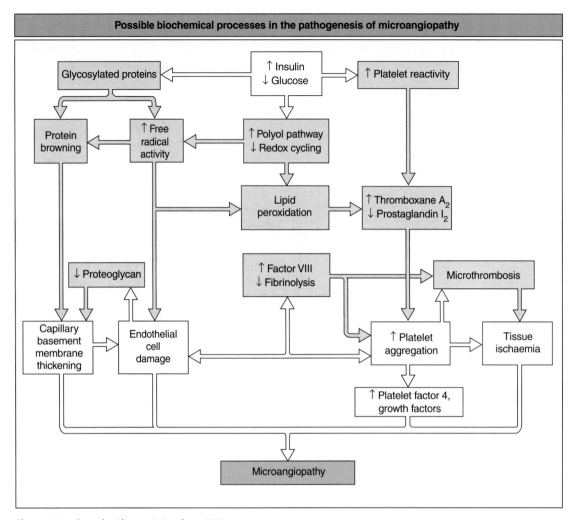

Figure 2.5. Adapted with permission from [26].

Diabetic retinopathy

Several studies have suggested that patients with diabetes and hypertension may be at a higher risk of developing particularly severe retinopathy compared with normotensive patients. There are reports of an association between hypertension and hard exudates, haemorrhages and other severe forms of retinopathy (Figures 2.7 and 2.8) [33–35] and some studies have found a relationship between proliferative retinopathy and elevated blood pressure (Figures 2.9 and 2.10) [36,37]. Both cross-sectional [38,39] and prospective studies [40] have indicated a particular role for progression of retinopathy. For example, the Pima Indian study prospectively analysed the relationship between blood pressure and retinopathy [40]. Pima Indians

of Arizona, USA have the world's largest reported incidence of type 2 diabetes, the peak being in early adulthood. Over a five-year period it was found that the incidence of retinal exudates in patients with diabetes and systolic blood pressure over 145 mmHg was more than twice that of patients whose systolic blood pressure was less than 125 mmHg. The study, however, found no relationship between blood pressure and retinal haemorrhages. More recent studies also support the contention that hypertension is a significant risk factor for diabetic retinopathy [41–43].

To date, there have been no prospective reports for type 1 diabetes, although retrospective studies suggest a high incidence of hypertension in patients with type 1 diabetes and retinopathy compared with

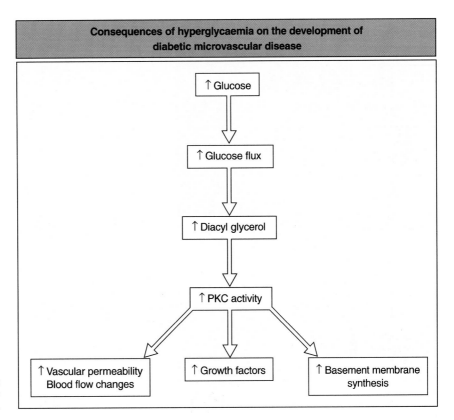

Figure 2.6. PKC, protein kinase C. Adapted with permission from [28].

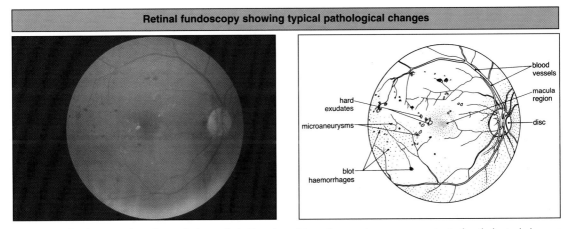

Figure 2.7. The disc, vessels and macula (central, dark) region of the retina can be seen, as can typical pathological changes of the retina: microaneurysms, hard exudates and haemorrhage.

matched patients without hypertension [44,45]. Another study investigated patients with type 1 diabetes who had been free of retinopathy for 30 years and found that factors protective against retinopathy included lower diastolic blood pressure at the time of analysis. Blood pressure did not, however, differ sig-nificantly between those patients with long-standing diabetes who were free of complications and matched patients with complications before the development of retinopathy, suggesting that there was no influence of blood pressure on the develop-ment of retinopathy [46].

Macular fundoscopy

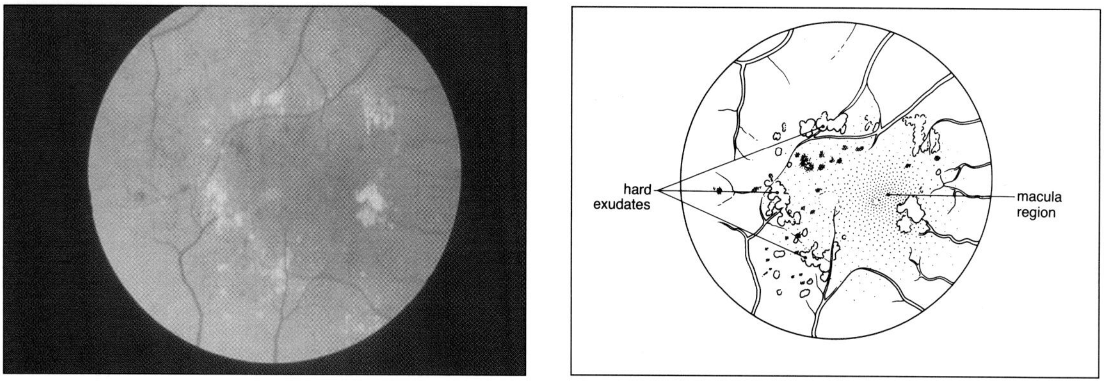

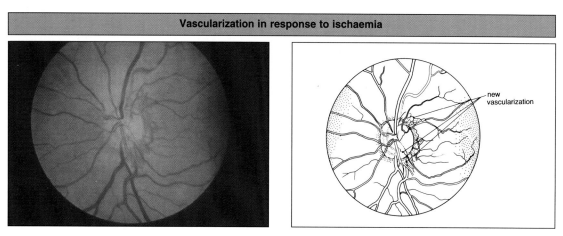

Figure 2.8. The macula is the light-gathering region of the retina. The development of rings of hard exudate suggests macular oedema and requires treatment.

Vascularization in response to ischaemia

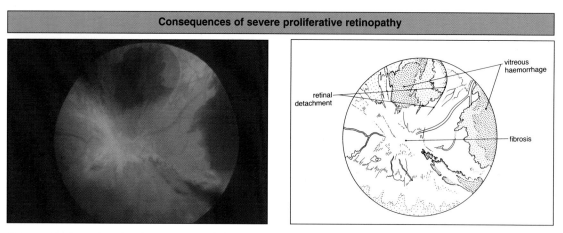

Figure 2.9. The growth of new vessels is from above the optic disc into the vitreous. These vessels form in response to ischaemia. If not treated appropriately (with laser), they are likely to bleed and may cause blindness.

Consequences of severe proliferative retinopathy

Figure 2.10. The end results of retinopathy include vitreous haemorrhage, fibrosis and retinal detachment. The eye is blind and beyond treatment.

The mechanism for progression of diabetic retinopathy in hypertension is not clear, but a 1995 study of experimental hypertension in humans demonstrated an impairment in retinal vascular autoregulation in response to raised systemic blood pressure in patients with diabetes, particularly in the presence of elevated blood glucose [47].

In conclusion, it is likely, but not yet firmly established, that hypertension plays a causative role in the development of retinopathy. Hypertension also appears to have a significant role in its progression.

Diabetic nephropathy

Hypertension is the single most important risk factor for progression of diabetic nephropathy and some believe it may even be an initiating factor. A genetic predisposition to hypertension appears to be associated with diabetic nephropathy even when systolic blood pressure is not raised. Other risk factors for development of nephropathy undoubtedly include poor glycaemic control. Diabetic nephropathy is considered in detail in Chapter 3.

Other microvascular complications

It is likely that both metabolic and microangiopathic factors are involved in the development of neuropathy (Figures 2.11–2.13). To date, no studies have specifically examined the link between hypertension and neuropathy. Other complications may include the specific heart muscle disease of diabetes, diabetic cardiomyopathy. Data suggest that myocardial dysfunction may be associated with diabetes in the absence of extensive coronary atherosclerosis [48]. Various studies have suggested small vessel (intramural) coronary artery disease, interstitial myocardial accumulation of glycoprotein and collagen, and metabolic alterations of the diabetic myocardium [49,50]. In an autopsy study of nine patients with diabetes who had clinically severe congestive heart failure and minimal extramural coronary atherosclerosis, all had hypertension. Severe interstitial fibrosis, focal or confluent scars and extensive myocytolytic activity were found more commonly in diabetic patients with hypertension when compared with patients who were without diabetes, normotensive with diabetes and hypertensive without diabetes [49]. The whole area of diabetic cardiomyopathy needs further clarification.

Diabetic neuropathic ulcer

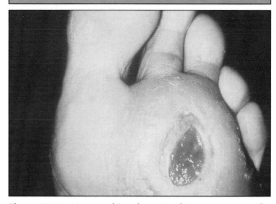

Figure 2.11. Neuropathic ulcers tend to occur over the weight-bearing areas of the foot, such as the metatarsal heads and tips of the toes, and are usually painless. They are often associated with much callous formation (removal in this case was by a chiropodist) and are usually well defined.

Inadequately treated neuropathic ulcer

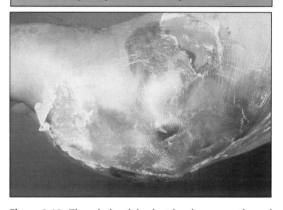

Figure 2.12. The whole of the foot has become a 'bag of pus'. The soft tissue as well as the underlying bone has become infected. There is pus dripping from an ulcer on the underside of the foot.

Effects of antihypertensive treatment in the patient with diabetes

The prevalence of hypertension in the population with diabetes is high, thus adding significantly to the risk of development and progression of both large and small vessel diseases. Since hypertension is such a powerful factor for vascular disease, it was assumed that lowering blood pressure would be of benefit. There was until recently no hard evidence for this, but a number of major trials have now been reported showing that aggressive

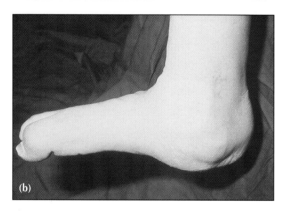

Charcot joints

Figure 2.13. Charcot joints: posterior (a) and lateral (b) views. This occasional complication of diabetic neuropathy is caused by a combination of (usually minor) trauma, severe neuropathy and localized osteoporosis. The joint has become completely deranged and ankylosed. Such feet are prone to further ulcer development and infection, and may eventually lead to major amputation of the limb.

control of blood pressure is vital in patients with diabetes.

Details of these studies can be found in Chapter 5 and are reviewed in [51]. One of the most important studies was the UKPDS substudy, the Hypertension in Diabetes Study (HDS). This nine-year study demonstrated that intensive treatment compared with conventional treatment of hypertension was associated with significant risk reductions for any diabetes-related end point, diabetes-related death,

fatal and non-fatal stroke, congestive heart failure and microvascular complications [52]. In addition, the Hypertension Optimal Treatment (HOT) study demonstrated a significant 51% reduction in major cardiovascular events in patients randomly allocated to the group given the target diastolic blood pressure of below 80 mmHg compared with a group where the target diastolic blood pressure was below 90 mmHg [53]. In both studies more than one antihypertensive agent was required in the majority of patients to achieve target blood pressures. The HOT study also provided the first evidence for the benefit of low-dose aspirin in patients with hypertension, with a significant reduction in major cardiovascular events, particularly myocardial infarction (reduction of 36%).

There is now also a wealth of data on the benefits of blood pressure lowering in diabetic microvascular disease, particularly nephropathy (*see* Chapter 3) and also in retinopathy [40,52,54].

Based on these important studies, new BHS guidelines not only stress the importance of aggressive treatment and management of hypertension in patients with diabetes, but also suggest much lower thresholds for intervention and treatment in these patients compared with previous recommendations [55]. These various trials and new guidelines are discussed in more detail in Chapter 5.

Summary

Hypertension is a major risk factor for diabetic vascular disease, both small and large vessel. Evidence now available demonstrates unequivocally that the lowering of blood pressure in diabetic patients with hypertension is associated with reduced risk of cardiovascular disease and cardiovascular mortality, and reduced risk of microvascular disease, including retinopathy and nephropathy. The treatment of hypertension in patients with diabetes is therefore clearly beneficial and recent guidelines suggest that hypertension should be screened for and treated aggressively in patients with diabetes, with lower thresholds for both intervention and treatment than previously recommended.

References

1. Anonymous. **Statement on hypertension in diabetes: final report. The Working Group on Hypertension in Diabetes.** *Arch Intern Med* 1987, **147**:830–842.

2. Barnett AH. **Diabetes and hypertension.** *Br Med Bull* 1994, **50**:397–407.

3. Kannel WB, McGee DL. **Diabetes and cardiovascular risk factors: the Framingham study.** *Circulation* 1979, **59**:8–13.

4. Stamler J. **Atherosclerotic coronary heart disease.** In *Diabetes Mellitus. Fourth edition.* Edited by KE Sussman and RJS Metz. New York: American Diabetes Association, 1975;229–241.

5. Goodkin G. **Mortality factors in diabetes. A 20 year mortality study.** *J Occup Med* 1975, **17**:716–721.

6. Kannel WB. **Some lessons in cardiovascular epidemiology from Framingham.** *Am J Cardiol* 1976, **37**: 269–282.

7. White P. **Natural course and prognosis of juvenile diabetes.** *Diabetes* 1956, **5**:445–450.

8. Deckert T, Poulsen JE, Larsen M. **Prognosis of diabetics with diabetes onset before the age of thirty-one. I. Survival, causes of death, and complications.** *Diabetologia* 1978, **14**:363–370.

9. Tunbridge WM. **Factors contributing to deaths of diabetics under fifty years of age. On behalf of the Medical Services Study Group and British Diabetic Association.** *Lancet* 1981, **2**:569–572.

10. Pell S, D'Alonzo CA. **Factors associated with long-term survival of diabetics.** *JAMA* 1970, **214**:1833–1840.

11. Keen H, Jarrett RJ, Fuller JH *et al.* **Hyperglycaemia and arterial disease.** *Diabetes* 1981, **30** (suppl. 2):49–53.

12. Tzagournis M. **Interaction of diabetes with hypertension and lipids—patients at high risk. An overview.** *Am J Med* 1989, **86**:50–54.

13. Maxwell SRJ, Barnett AH. **The management of hypertension in the diabetic patient** In *Difficult Hypertension.* Edited by MJ Kendall, NM Kaplan and RC Horton. London: Martin Dunitz, 1995;135–160.

14. Roehmholdt ME, Palumbo PJ, Whisnant JP *et al.* **Transient ischaemic attack and stroke in a community-based diabetic cohort.** *Mayo Clin Proc* 1983, **58**: 56–58.

15. Kuller LH, Dorman JS, Wolf PA. **Cerebrovascular disease and diabetes.** In *Diabetes in America (85-1468).* Washington, DC: US Department of Health and Human Services, 1985;1–8.

16. Palumbo PJ, Elveback LR, Whisnant JP. **Neurologic complications of diabetes mellitus: transient ischaemic attack, stroke, and peripheral neuropathy.** *Adv Neurol* 1978, **19**:593–601.

17. Bell D. **Stroke in the diabetic patient.** *Diabetes Care* 1994, **17**:213–219.

18. Asplund K, Hägg E, Helmers C *et al.* **The natural history of stroke in diabetic patients.** *Acta Med Scand* 1980, **207**:417–424.

19. Janka HV, Standl E, Mehnert H. **Peripheral vascular disease in diabetes mellitus and its relation to cardiovascular risk factors: screening with the doppler ultrasonic technique.** *Diabetes Care* 1980, **3**:207–213.

20. Baird RN. **Distensibility of the arterial wall in diabetes.** In *Hormones and Vascular Disease.* Edited by RM Greenhalf. London: Pitman Medical, 1981;139–142.

21. McMillan DE. **Physical factors important in the development of atherosclerosis in diabetes.** *Diabetes* 1981, **30** (suppl. 2):97–104.

22. Pirart J. **[Diabetes mellitus and its degenerative complications: a prospective study of 4,400 patients observed between 1947 and 1973 (2nd part).]** *Diabete Metab* 1977, **3**:173–182.

23. Tchobroutsky G. **Relation of diabetic control to development of microvascular complications.** *Diabetologia* 1978, **15**:143–152.

24. Skyler JS. **Complications of diabetes mellitus: relationship to metabolic dysfunction.** *Diabetes Care* 1979, **2**:498–509.

25. Tooke JE. **The microcirculation in diabetes.** *Diabet Med* 1987, **4**:189–196.

26. Jennings PE, Barnett AH. **New approaches to the pathogenesis and treatment of diabetic microangiopathy.** *Diabet Med* 1988, **5**:111–117.

27. Brownlee M, Vlassara H, Cerami A. **Nonenzymatic glycosylation and the pathogenesis of diabetic complications.** *Ann Intern Med* 1984, **101**:527–537.

28. Giardino I, Brownlee M. **The biochemical basis of microvascular disease.** In *Textbook of Diabetes. Second edition.* Edited by JC Pickup and G Williams. Oxford: Blackwell Science Ltd, 1996;16.

29. Cogan DG, Kinoshita JH, Kador PF *et al.* **NIH conference. Aldose reductase and complications of diabetes.** *Ann Intern Med* 1984, **101**:82–91.

30. Grant M, Russell B, Fitzgerald C *et al.* **Insulin-like growth factors in vitreous studies in control and diabetic subjects with neovascularisation.** *Diabetes* 1986, **35**: 416–420.

31. Koya D, King GL. **Protein kinase C activation and the development of diabetic complications.** *Diabetes* 1998, **47**:859–866.

32. Giardino I, Edelstein D, Brownlee M. **Nonenzymatic glycosylation *in vitro* and in bovine endothelial cells alters basic fibroblast growth factor activity. A model for intracellular glycosylation in diabetes.** *J Clin Invest* 1994, **94**:110–117.

33. Fuller JH. **Blood pressure and diabetes mellitus.** In *Epidemiology of Hypertension.* Edited by CJ Bulpitt. Amsterdam: Elsevier, 1985;318–330.

34. Kornerup T. **Blood pressure and diabetic retinopathy.** *Acta Ophthalmol* 1957, **35**:163–174.

35. Chahal P, Inglesby DV, Sleightholm M *et al.* **Blood pressure and the progression of mild background diabetic retinopathy.** *Hypertension* 1985, **7** (suppl. 2):79–83.

36. Klein R, Klein BE, Moss SE *et al.* **The Wisconsin epidemiologic study of diabetic retinopathy. II. Prevalence and risk of diabetic retinopathy when age at diagnosis is less than 30 years.** *Arch Ophthalmol* 1984, **102**:520–526.

37. Klein R, Klein BE, Moss SE *et al.* **The Wisconsin epidemiologic study of diabetic retinopathy. III. Prevalence and risk factors of diabetic retinopathy when age at diagnosis is 30 or more years.** *Arch Ophthalmol* 1984, **102**:527–532.

38. Barnett AH, Britton JR, Leatherdale BA. **Study of possible risk factors for severe retinopathy in non-insulin dependent diabetes.** *Br Med J (Clin Res Ed)* 1983, **287**:529.

39. Mouton DP, Gill AJ. **Prevalence of diabetic retinopathy and evaluation of risk factors. A review of 1,005 diabetic clinic patients.** *S Afr Med J* 1988, **74**:399–402.

40. Knowler WC, Bennett PH, Ballintine EJ. **Increased incidence of retinopathy in diabetics with elevated blood pressure. A six-year follow-up study in Pima Indians.** *N Engl J Med* 1980, **302**:645–650.

41. Lewis JM, Jovanovic-Peterson L, Ahmadizadeh I *et al.* **The Santa Barbara County diabetic retinopathy screening feasibility study: significance of diabetes duration and systolic blood pressure.** *J Diabetes Complications* 1994, **8**:51–54.

42. Cignarelli M, De Cicco ML, Damato A *et al.* **High systolic blood pressure increases prevalence and severity of retinopathy in NIDDM patients.** *Diabetes Care* 1992, **15**:1002–1008.

43. Dodson PM, Gibson JM. **Long-term follow-up of and underlying medical conditions in patients with diabetic exudative maculopathy.** *Eye* 1991, **5**:699–703.

44. Drury PL. **Diabetes and arterial hypertension.** *Diabetologia* 1983, **24**:1–9.

45. Drury PL, Bodansky H, Oddie CJ et al. **Increased plasma renin activity in type 1 diabetes with microvascular diseases.** *Clin Endocrinol (Oxf)* 1982, **16**:453–461.

46. Dornan T, Mann JI, Turner R. **Factors protective against retinopathy in insulin-dependent diabetics free of retinopathy for 30 years.** *Br Med J* 1982, **285**:1073–1077.

47. Rassam SM, Patel V, Kohner EM. **The effect of experimental hypertension on retinal vascular autoregulation in humans: a mechanism for progression of diabetic retinopathy.** *Exp Physiol* 1995, **80**:53–68.

48. Regan TJ, Weisse AJB. **The question of cardiomyopathy in diabetes mellitus.** *Ann Intern Med* 1978, **89**:1000–1002.

49. Factor SM, Minase T, Sonnenblick EH. **Clinical and morphological features of human hypertensive diabetic cardiomyopathy.** *Am Heart J* 1980, **99**:446–458.

50. van Hoeven KH, Factor SM. **The diabetic heart: clinical, experimental and pathological features.** *Acta Cardiol* 1991, **46**:329–339.

51. Chowdhury TA, Kumar S, Barnett AH *et al.* **Treatment of hypertension in patients with type 2 diabetes: a review of the recent evidence.** *J Hum Hypertens* 1999, **13**:803–811.

52. Anonymous. **Tight blood pressure control and risk of macrovascular and microvascular complications in type 2 diabetes: UKPDS 38. United Kingdom Prospective Diabetes Study Group.** *Br Med J* 1998, **317**:703–713.

53. Hansson L, Zanchetti A, Carruthers SG *et al.* **Effects of intensive blood pressure lowering and low-dose aspirin in patients with hypertension: principal results of the Hypertension Optimal Treatment (HOT) randomised trial. HOT Study Group.** *Lancet* 1998, **351**:1755–1762.

54. Gillow JT, Gibson JM, Dodson PM. **Hypertension and diabetic retinopathy – what's the story?** *Br J Ophthalmol* 1999, **83**:1083–1087.

55. Ramsay LE, Williams B, Johnston GD *et al.* **British Hypertension Society guidelines for hypertension management 1999: summary.** *Br Med J* 1999, **319**:630–635.

Hypertension and nephropathy in diabetes

Diabetic nephropathy comprises proteinuria, hypertension and declining renal function. The onset of nephropathy not only indicates an increased renal morbidity, but also a dramatic increase in cardiovascular mortality [1]. This chapter reviews the role of hypertension in the development and progression of diabetic nephropathy and the ways in which treatment of hypertension may affect its progression.

Epidemiology and prevalence

Early studies suggest that approximately 30% of patients with diabetes develop nephropathy [2], although more recent studies suggest that the incidence is now lower, possibly because of improvements in metabolic control [3]. Increased risk of nephropathy is seen in men and in Asian and Afro-Caribbean populations [4].

In the UK, diabetic nephropathy accounts for around 600 cases of end-stage renal failure (ESRF) per year [5]. Patients with nephropathy have a relative mortality 40–100 times that of patients without diabetes [6]. After the onset of persistent proteinuria, survival after five years is around 65%; at 10 years this is only 28% [7]. Recent statistics suggest an improved prognosis in diabetic nephropathy to around 82% for 10-year survival, probably because of improvements in blood pressure therapy [3].

Stages of diabetic nephropathy

Albuminuria is the hallmark of diabetic renal disease. The first phase is microalbuminuria, defined as an albumin excretion rate (AER) above the normal range but below the level of detection of reagent strips that detect protein in urine (20–200 μg/min [30–300 mg/24 hours]). Incipient nephropathy is regarded as present if two out of three urine samples examined within a six-month period show microalbuminuria. This incipient nephropathy phase is rare if the duration of diabetes is less than five years.

Macroalbuminuria is the excretion of albumin detectable by protein reagent strips. If retinopathy is untreated, ESRF usually occurs within 10 years. Approximately 80% of patients with microalbuminuria progress to overt nephropathy within 10 years [8], although a 1994 prospective study suggested that the figure is around 40% [9]. In type 2 diabetes, microalbuminuria is less consistently linked with progression of overt nephropathy, but is associated with an increase in cardiovascular disease [10]. Mogensen has proposed a scheme dividing diabetic nephropathy into five stages (Table 3.1).

Stage 1: Glomerular hyperfunction and hypertrophy. These changes are present at diagnosis of diabetes. The glomerular filtration rate (GFR) is raised and blood pressure is normal (Figure 3.1).

Stage 2: Normal AER and normal, or only slightly increased, blood pressure. Hyperfiltration in the kidney may be present. Structural abnormalities (basement membrane thickening) are present at this stage.

Stage 3: Incipient nephropathy. There is a persistent degree of microalbuminuria. Blood pressure is often elevated compared with healthy subjects

Stages of diabetic nephropathy				
Stage	Characteristics	Albumin excretion rate	Glomerular filtration rate	Blood pressure
1	Hypertrophy and hyperfunction	Normal	Raised	Normal
2	Abnormal structure	Normal	Raised or normal	Normal or slightly elevated
3	Persistent microproteinuria	20–200 μg/min	Raised, normal or low	Raised compared with normal subjects
4	Macroproteinuria	>200 μg/min	Low	Frank hypertension
5	Uraemia	High or low	<10 ml/min	Hypertension

Table 3.1

Glomerular structure in early diabetic nephropathy

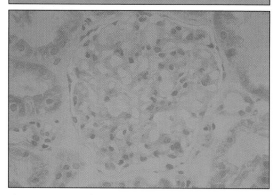

Figure 3.1. Histology section (haemotoxylin and eosin stained) of a kidney biopsy from a patient with early nephropathy, which shows no structural abnormalities.

and there is a loss of diurnal variation (non-dipping).

Stage 4: Overt diabetic nephropathy. There is persistent (Albustix-positive) proteinuria with hypertension and a decline in GFR.

Stage 5: ESRF with uraemia. This stage requires treatment by dialysis or transplantation (Figure 3.2).

Factors involved in the development of diabetic nephropathy

Diabetic nephropathy is associated with an increased risk of death and morbidity from microvascular and macrovascular disease [11]. The Saint Vincent declaration suggested that a

Glomerular changes typical of late diabetic nephropathy

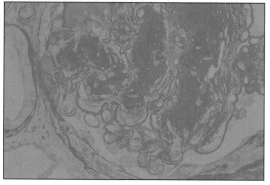

Figure 3.2. Histology section (haemotoxylin and eosin stained) of a renal biopsy from a patient with long-standing diabetes and diabetic nephropathy showing almost complete glomerulosclerosis.

decrease of a third in the incidence of ESRF in patients with diabetes was an achievable goal [12]. Prevention of diabetic nephropathy assumes an understanding of the pathophysiological processes involved in its development and the availability of effective means of influencing them.

Factors that are important in the development of diabetic nephropathy are hereditary factors, metabolic control and blood pressure control.

Hereditary factors

Diabetic nephropathy, particularly in type 1 diabetes, appears to have a considerable genetic influence in its aetiology. A number of observations support this:

- early studies suggested that the maximum prevalence of nephropathy is around 40%, despite patients in these early studies having poor glycaemic control [2];

- the incidence of nephropathy appears to increase up to 15 years from diagnosis of diabetes, then rapidly declines [2]. This contrasts sharply with other microangiopathic complications, which appear to increase in incidence with duration of diabetes;

- two studies have shown familial clustering of nephropathy in type 1 diabetes. Thus, in families with two children with diabetes, if one child develops nephropathy the second child has a four-fold increased risk of developing it [13,14]; and

- epidemiological studies suggest that offspring with diabetes have a much greater risk of developing nephropathy if their parents have hypertension [15], or have cardiovascular disease [16], than if their parents have neither.

The gene or genes involved in this process have yet to be characterized. Genes involved in the susceptibility to hypertension or cardiovascular disease are suitable candidates, including genes of the RAS. Genes encoding components of the RAS, including ACE, have been studied, but appear to have no major influence on the development of nephropathy [17]. It appears, however, that this genetic polymorphism may influence the response to treatment with ACE inhibitor drugs, with certain genotypes being more responsive to the renoprotective effects of ACE inhibitors than others [18]. Other genetic loci implicated in the pathogenesis of the condition include aldose reductase [19], and apolipoprotein E [20]. A genetic marker for nephropathy would enable patients to be screened on diagnosis of diabetes for increased risk of nephropathy; early initiation of treatment may be a possibility in the future.

Metabolic control

Diabetic nephropathy only develops in the presence of diabetes. Until recently, the only evidence to back-up claims that the level of glycaemia influences the onset of nephropathy was from small non-randomized studies [21]. The Diabetes Control and Complications Trial (DCCT) adds weight to the argument that metabolic factors are important [22]. Intensive treatment of glycaemia in type 1 diabetes appears to reduce the onset of microalbuminuria by around 60% compared with conventionally treated patients. Interestingly, subsequent analysis of the DCCT cohorts indicates that in patients with microalbuminuria, an improvement in glycaemic control does not stop the progression of incipient nephropathy to overt nephropathy, suggesting that microalbuminuria may represent an advanced stage of nephropathy [23].

Results of the recent UKPDS [24] have shown that metabolic control can influence nephropathy in type 2 diabetes, with a significant reduction in progression to microalbuminuria or macroalbuminuria in patients with tight blood glucose control, as compared with those with less tight glucose control.

Blood pressure control

There is considerable evidence to suggest that hypertension plays a pivotal role in the development and progression of diabetic nephropathy and, moreover, that lowering blood pressure may affect the rate of disease progression.

Aetiology of hypertension in diabetic nephropathy

There is a correlation between mean arterial pressure and AER in individuals with and without diabetes, although patients with diabetes have much higher AERs [25]. These higher AERs cause hypertension in most patients with diabetic nephropathy. The aetiology of this type of hypertension has yet to be fully determined, but is almost certainly multi-factorial and dependent upon genetic disturbance (*see* above) and hormonal disturbance.

Diabetic patients with hypertension have increased plasma volume caused by increased exchangeable body sodium. These changes may occur before the onset of hypertension [26]. The increased exchangeable sodium is further exacerbated by the onset of nephropathy [27]. The reason for the high levels of exchangeable sodium is not known, although insulin has been shown to promote renal tubular reabsorption of sodium [28]. The increase in body sodium leads to fluid retention and plasma volume expansion, thus favouring the development of hypertension.

The RAS plays a central role in the regulation of vascular tone and sodium–water homeostasis (Figure 3.3). Overactivation of the RAS is seen in diabetic nephropathy. Plasma renin activity, serum ACE activity and plasma prorenin levels are all higher in nephropathic individuals [29]. Furthermore, patients with diabetes have an enhanced pressor response to infused angiotensin II [30], possibly owing to elevated numbers of the angiotensin II receptor [31]. This may lead to enhanced effects from circulating angiotensin II and predispose to glomerular hyperfiltration.

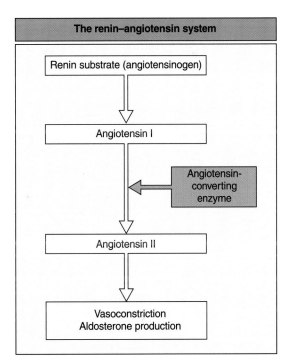

Figure 3.3

Glomerular hypertension and diabetic nephropathy

Glomerular hyperfiltration appears to be a risk factor for the development of diabetic nephropathy (Figure 3.4) [32,33]. Patients with diabetes and persistent hyperfiltration are more likely to progress to overt nephropathy than patients with lower initial GFR [34]. Filtration at the glomerulus is dependent on the intrinsic permeability of the glomerular basement membrane, which in turn is determined by pore size and electrical charge. Loss of heparan sulphate, a negatively charged proteoglycan, from the base-ment membrane accounts for its loss of permselec-tivity, hence leading to urinary protein loss [35]. Filtration is also affected by renal perfusion and intracapillary pressure. Unilateral nephrectomy appears to accelerate diabetic nephropathy by increasing glomerular perfusion in the remaining kidney [36]. Studies in rats with diabetes indicate that lowering intraglomerular pressure using ACE inhibitors prevents the onset of nephropathy, which suggests intraglomerular hypertension is influential in the development of nephropathy [37].

Hypertension in incipient diabetic nephropathy

Interest has recently focused on the possibility of treating patients at an earlier stage of nephropathy, to stop its progression. Incipient nephropathy may last up to 15 years before it progresses to overt

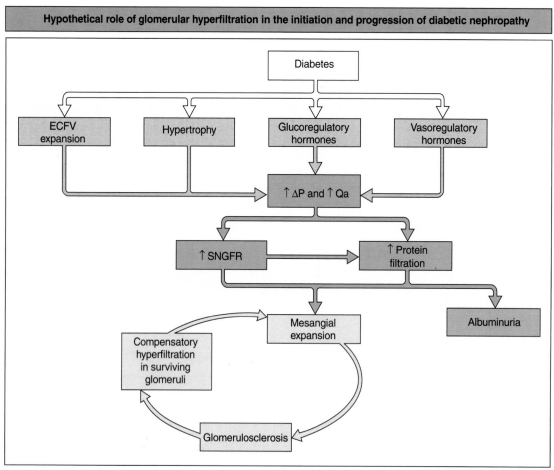

Hypothetical role of glomerular hyperfiltration in the initiation and progression of diabetic nephropathy

Figure 3.4. Hyperfiltration is stimulated by extracellular fluid volume (ECFV) expansion, renal hypertrophy and/or vasoactive hormones. Increases in the glomerular transcapillary hydraulic pressure gradient (ΔP) and glomerular plasma flow rate (Qa) are responsible for hyperfiltration leading to albuminuria, mesangial deposition of circulating proteins and ultimately, glomerulosclerosis. Loss of functioning nephrons exerts a positive-feedback stimulus to compensatory hyperfiltration in surviving glomeruli, thus contributing to their destruction. SNGFR, single-nephron glomerular filtration rate. Reprinted with permission from [32].

nephropathy, although around 60% of patients with microalbuminuria may never progress that far [9].

A number of studies suggest that treatment of blood pressure in incipient nephropathy delays progression of the condition. Early small studies have shown a decrease in the rate of the progressive rise of AER with combined beta-blocker and diuretic therapy [38]. Larger prospective studies have shown that antihypertensive therapy with ACE inhibitors in patients with microalbuminuria appears to protect against the development of overt nephropathy. In one multicentre, double-blind, randomized, parallel group study, 335 patients with type 2 diabetes and microalbuminuria were examined. The patients were randomly allocated to groups that received treatment with either lisinopril or nifedipine [39]. Blood pressure and glycaemic control in the two treatment groups were not significantly different over the one-year study period. A significant reduction in urine albumin excretion was, however, seen in the lisinopril-treated group over the year.

In type 1 diabetes, a number of small studies have examined hypertensive patients with microalbuminuria. The Melbourne Diabetic Nephropathy Study Group examined 43 patients with microalbuminuria and found that treatment of blood pressure with either perindopril or nifedipine caused a reduction in the progressive rise of AER after one year with no significant difference in efficacy between the two treatment groups [40]. Hallab and colleagues conducted a similar randomized, double-blind study of 21 patients with microalbuminuria comparing enalapril with hydrochlorothiazide [41]. Blood pressure control was similar in both groups, but reduction in AER was significantly greater in the enalapril-treated group. Although these studies suggest that blood pressure control appears to be beneficial in preventing the rise in AER in patients with microalbuminuria, longer-term follow-up is required to see whether these beneficial effects persist.

The question arises as to whether antihypertensive therapy in normotensive patients with microalbuminuria delays or prevents the onset of established nephropathy. Although patients with microalbuminuria are commonly normotensive as defined by the WHO criteria, they have blunting of diurnal blood pressure variation and slightly elevated blood pressure compared with age-matched control subjects. As these patients often develop hypertension, early therapy to achieve a modest reduction in blood pressure may prevent the onset of overt nephropathy. The results of a placebo-controlled trial of captopril-treated patients with normotension, microalbuminuria and type 1 diabetes, showed a significant reduction in AER in the treated group [42]. Similar results have been seen with enalapril versus placebo; after one year, 30% of the placebo-treated group developed nephropathy compared with none in the enalapril-treated group, of whom 50% reverted to normo-albuminuria [43]. A recent larger study of 490 patients with type 1 diabetes and normoalbuminuria or microalbuminuria found that treatment with lisinopril reduced microalbuminuria by 49.7% [39].

Although not fully established, it appears that the treatment of patients who have microalbuminuria and normotension or microalbuminuria and mild hypertension, with antihypertensive therapy is of benefit in reduction of progression to overt nephropathy. A number of studies suggest that ACE inhibitors are of particular benefit in such patients.

Treatment of hypertension and prevention of diabetic nephropathy

Does treatment of hypertension delay the onset of nephropathy in patients with diabetes? This question has been addressed, in patients with type 2 diabetes, by the blood pressure arm of the UKPDS [44]. This study compared tight blood pressure control (target blood pressure <150/85 mmHg; n=758) with standard blood pressure control (target blood pressure <180/105 mmHg; n=390). The blood pressures achieved were 144/82 mmHg and 155/87 mmHg, respectively; death from myocardial infarction was reduced by 21%, the incidence of stroke was reduced by 44% and overall microvascular disease was reduced by 34% in the tight blood pressure control group. Elevation of the urinary AER to greater than 50 mg/l and greater than 300 mg/l was reduced by 29% and 39%, respectively, in the tight control group.

This suggests that treatment of hypertension in patients with type 2 diabetes can delay or prevent the onset of nephropathy.

Hypertension in overt diabetic nephropathy

Hypertension is associated with diabetic nephropathy and plays a role in its development. Patients with persistent hypertension have a faster decline in renal function compared with normotensive patients.

Small, early studies of antihypertensive therapy in diabetic nephropathy suggested that treatment slows, but does not stop, the decline into ESRF [45]. A significant reduction in the decline of GFR could be achieved with vigorous antihypertensive therapy using a wide variety of agents in patients with diabetes (Figure 3.5) [46]. The decline of renal function could not, however, be completely stopped.

Lewis *et al* [47] studied the effect of the ACE inhibitor, captopril, in patients with type 1 diabetes. Captopril provided protection against deterioration

in renal function and was more effective than blood pressure control alone in this study. An extension to this study [48] has shown that a combination of ACE inhibition and intensive blood pressure control can result in regression of clinical signs of diabetic nephropathy.

Long-term follow up of patients with persistent proteinuria and treated hypertension has shown a dramatic decline in the cumulative death rate caused by diabetic nephropathy, to around 18%, 10 years after onset; overall mortality was 31% [3]. These results are in marked contrast to previous reports of death rates between 50% and 77% over a similar time period [7].

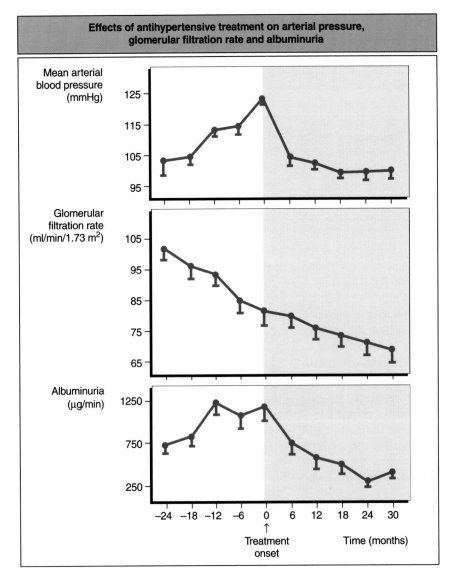

Effects of antihypertensive treatment on arterial pressure, glomerular filtration rate and albuminuria

Figure 3.5. Reprinted with permission from [46].

Influence of hypertension on cardiovascular mortality in diabetic nephropathy

Patients with type 1 diabetes who develop persistent proteinuria have an increased mortality compared with patients who have normoalbuminuria. This is predominantly caused by an excess cardiovascular mortality. Hypertension is an important contributory factor to cardiovascular deaths in patients with ESRF [49]. A retrospective analysis of patient and graft survival showed that hypertension is closely linked with survival of both grafts and patients receiving renal transplants [50].

Hypertension and pregnancy in diabetic nephropathy

A population-based study found that the incidence of nephropathy was 3.8% in pregnant women with diabetes [51]. Hypertension is a common complication of diabetes and may worsen during pregnancy. Proteinuria may also increase, but returns to pre-pregnancy levels following delivery. Deterioration in renal function may occur after pregnancy but appears to be compatible with the natural history of nephropathy itself, rather than as a consequence of pregnancy. Women with severe renal disease (regardless of aetiology) rarely conceive. Worsening hypertension in the third trimester with an accompanying increase in proteinuria is difficult to distinguish from pre-eclampsia, as there are no reliable discriminatory laboratory tests. Although a planned pregnancy is more likely to have a successful outcome, treatment should ideally begin before conception, with advice regarding contraception, diet, exercise and strict metabolic control.

When pregnancy is confirmed, meticulous attention must be paid to control of blood glucose and blood pressure levels. Women who become nephrotic may require diuretics, although methyldopa is a well-established drug for blood pressure control in pregnancy. Beta-blockers (atenolol and oxprenolol) have been used in clinical trials and used extensively in clinical practice without serious adverse effects for mother or fetus; other frequently used drugs are hydralazine and labetolol. ACE inhibitors are contraindicated during pregnancy. Available data suggest that their use carries a risk of early delivery, low birth weight and oligohydramnios and neonatal anuria in the children born [52].

Treatment of hypertension in diabetic nephropathy

The British Hypertension Society guidelines

As a result of new clinical evidence, a number of BHS guidelines have been published suggesting thresholds and targets for antihypertensive therapy in patients with diabetes [53]. The recommendations are summarized in Table 3.2 [53], which includes suggested thresholds and targets for patients with diabetic nephropathy.

Diuretics

Increased sodium levels in diabetic patients with hypertension means that they often respond well to initial treatment with a loop diuretic. Large doses may be required in those with advanced renal failure, particularly if fluid retention is present.

Beta-blockers

Beta-blockers were among the first drugs to be used in the treatment of diabetic nephropathy. Large-scale

British Hypertension Society guidelines on treating hypertension in patients with diabetes				
	Type 1 diabetes		Type 2 diabetes	
	Without nephropathy	With nephropathy	Without nephropathy	With nephropathy
Threshold for treatment (mmHg)	≥140/90	≥140/90	≥140/90	≥140/90
Target blood pressure (mmHg)	<140/80	<130/80*	<140/80	<130/85*

Table 3.2. *target blood pressure <125/75 mmHg, if proteinuria >1 g/day. Data from [53].

studies have demonstrated their cardioprotective properties in patients without diabetes who have sustained a heart attack. Patients with diabetic nephropathy have an increased cardiovascular mortality, but no studies have directly addressed whether beta-blockers are cardioprotective in these patients. Trials of beta-blockers in diabetic nephropathy have shown good results. In type 2 diabetes, beta-blockers produced a lesser reduction in albuminuria compared with ACE inhibitors, but a similar reduction in the rate of decline of GFR was seen [54]. In type 1 diabetes, comparison of a beta-blocker with an ACE inhibitor showed equivalent reductions in albuminuria and rate of decline of GFR [55]. Beta-blockers may alter the patient's awareness of hypoglycaemia, although influences on lipid and glycaemic profiles appear to be small.

Calcium antagonists

Calcium antagonists are useful agents in patients with diabetes as they do not affect metabolic control. In renal impairment, where fluid retention may be a problem, the tendency to cause pedal oedema may reduce their usefulness. A number of studies have compared calcium antagonists with other antihypertensive agents in patients with diabetic nephropathy. One study showed equivalent effects of perindopril and nifedipine in patients with microalbuminuria and type 1 diabetes [40], although a greater reduction in albuminuria in lisinopril-treated compared with nifedipine-treated patients has been observed in patients with type 2 diabetes [39]. It has been suggested that non-dihydropyridine calcium antagonists (diltiazem and verapamil) may offer greater renoprotection than dihydropyridine drugs (nifedipine), possibly because of differing effects on renal tubular function [56].

Angiotensin-converting enzyme inhibitors

ACE inhibitors are efficacious in the treatment of systemic hypertension and, as with other anti-hypertensive drugs, reduce proteinuria in diabetic nephropathy. ACE inhibitors exert their intra-renal effects predominantly at the efferent arteriole, causing vasodilatation and thus lowering intra-glomerular hypertension (Figure 3.6) [57]. Early studies showed that ACE inhibitors significantly reduced albuminuria and the rate of decline of GFR compared with placebo [58]. ACE inhibitors also appear to reduce incidence of death and ESRF

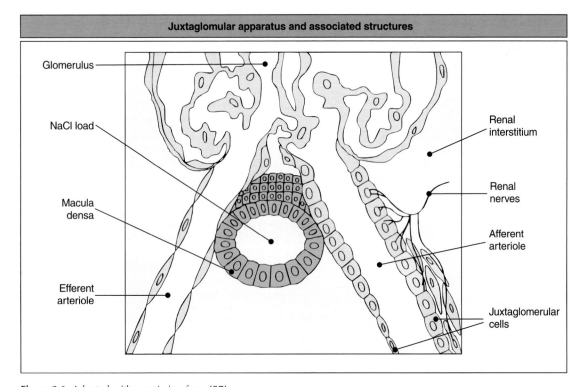

Juxtaglomular apparatus and associated structures

Glomerulus

NaCl load

Macula densa

Efferent arteriole

Renal interstitium

Renal nerves

Afferent arteriole

Juxtaglomerular cells

Figure 3.6. Adapted with permission from [57].

compared with placebo [59]. Comparison of ACE inhibitors with other anithypertensive agents suggests that they may have a beneficial effect over and above their antihypertensive effect. Comparison of enalapril and metoprolol in patients with type 1 diabetes and nephropathy showed a halving of the rate of decline of GFR in the enalapril-treated group, despite equivalent blood pressure [60]. As stated previously, studies comparing ACE inhibitors with calcium antagonists in patients with type 2 diabetes have yielded similar results [39].

Careful monitoring of renal function should be undertaken in all patients who begin ACE inhibitor therapy. Renal function should be checked before and shortly after commencing therapy to ensure that a sudden decline in renal function does not occur.

Summary

Hypertension is common in diabetic nephropathy, although whether it is a cause or a result of nephropathy is not, as yet, clear. Genetic factors, metabolic control and haemodynamic factors contribute to the development of nephropathy. Hypertension exacerbates nephropathy and may contribute to increased cardiovascular mortality. Control of hypertension slows the rate of decline of renal function and may stop proteinuria worsening. Although no drug has been shown to be consistently superior to others, ACE inhibitors show, in studies, a good tolerance and few side effects with a renoprotective effect over and above their antihypertensive effect. Recent investigation suggests that ACE inhibitors may be of value in preventing the onset of overt nephropathy in patients with incipient nephropathy. Further comparative and long-term studies are required to determine fully the role of ACE inhibitor drugs in the treatment of renal disease in patients with diabetes, particularly in type 2 diabetes.

References

1. Borch-Johnsen K, Andersen PK, Deckert T. **The effect of proteinuria on relative mortality in type 1 (insulin-dependent) diabetes mellitus**. *Diabetologia* 1985, **28**:590–596.

2. Anderson AR, Christiansen JS, Anderson JK *et al.* **Diabetic nephropathy in type I (insulin-dependent) diabetes: an epidemiological study**. *Diabetologia* 1983, **25**:496–501.

3. Parving HH, Hommel E. **Prognosis in diabetic nephropathy**. *Br Med J* 1989, **299**:230–233.

4. West KM, Edreich L, Stober JA. **A detailed study of risk factors for retinopathy and nephropathy in diabetes.** *Diabetes* 1980, **29**:501–508.

5. Anonymous. **Renal failure in diabetics in the UK: deficient provision of care in 1985. Joint Working Party on Diabetic Renal Failure of the British Diabetic Association, the Renal Association, and the Research Unit of the Royal College of Physicians.** *Diabet Med* 1988, **5**:79–84.

6. Caird FJ. **Survival of diabetics with proteinuria.** *Diabetes* 1961, **10**:178–181.

7. Krolewski AS, Warram JH, Christlieb AR *et al.* **The changing natural history of nephropathy in type 1 diabetes.** *Am J Med* 1985, **78**:785–794.

8. Viberti GC, Hill RD, Jarrett RJ *et al.* **Microalbuminuria as a predictor of clinical nephropathy in insulin-dependent diabetes mellitus.** *Lancet* 1982, **1**:1430–1432.

9. Almdal T, Nörgaard K, Feldt-Rasmussen B *et al.* **The predictive value of microalbuminuria in IDDM. A five-year follow-up study.** *Diabetes Care* 1994, **17**:120–125.

10. Yudkin JS, Forrest RD, Jackson CA. **Microalbuminuria as predictor of vascular disease in non-diabetic subjects. Islington Diabetes Survey.** *Lancet* 1988, **2**:530–533.

11. Deckert T, Feldt-Rasmussen B, Borch-Johnsen K *et al.* **Albuminuria reflects widespread vascular damage. The Steno hypothesis.** *Diabetologia* 1989, **32**:219–226.

12. Anonymous. **Diabetes care and research in Europe: the Saint Vincent declaration.** *Diabet Med* 1990, **7**:360.

13. Seaquist ER, Goetz FC, Rich S *et al.* **Familial clustering of diabetic kidney disease. Evidence for genetic susceptibility to diabetic nephropathy.** *N Engl J Med* 1989, **320**:1161–1165.

14. Borch-Johnsen K, Nørgaard K, Hommel E *et al.* **Is diabetic nephropathy an inherited complication?** *Kidney Int* 1992, **41**:719–722.

15. Viberti GC, Keen H, Wiseman MJ. **Raised arterial pressure in parents of proteinuric insulin-dependent diabetics.** *Br Med J* 1987, **295**:515–517.

16. Earle K, Walker J, Hill C *et al.* **Familial clustering of cardiovascular disease in patients with insulin-dependent diabetes and nephropathy.** *N Engl J Med* 1992, **326**:673–677.

17. Chowdhury TA, Dronsfield MJ, Kumar S *et al.* **Examination of two genetic polymorphisms within the renin–angiotensin system: no evidence for an association with nephropathy in IDDM.** *Diabetologia* 1996, **39**:1108–1114.

18. Parving HH, Jacobsen P, Tarnow L *et al.* **Effect of deletion polymorphism of angiotensin converting enzyme gene on progression of diabetic nephropathy during inhibition of angiotensin converting enzyme: observational follow up study.** *Br Med J* 1996, **313**:591–594.

19. Heesom AE, Hibberd ML, Millward A *et al.* **Polymorphism in the 5'-end of the aldose reductase gene is strongly associated with the development of diabetic nephropathy in type I diabetes.** *Diabetes* 1997, **46**: 287–291.

20. Chowdhury TA, Dyer PH, Kumar S *et al.* **Association of apolipoprotein ε2 allele with diabetic nephropathy in Caucasian subjects with IDDM.** *Diabetes* 1998, **47**:278–281.

21. Viberti GC, Bilous RW, Mackintosh D *et al.* **Long term correction of hyperglycaemia and progression of renal failure in insulin dependent diabetes.** *Br Med J* 1983, **286**:598–602.

22. Anonymous. **The effect of intensive treatment of diabetes on the development and progression of long-term complications in insulin-dependent diabetes mellitus. The Diabetes Control and Complication Research Group.** *N Engl J Med* 1993, **329**:977–986.

23. Anonymous. **Effect of intensive therapy on the development and progression of diabetic nephropathy in the Diabetes Control and Complications Trial. The Diabetes Control and Complications (DCCT) Research Group.** *Kidney Int* 1995, **47**:1703–1720.

24. Anonymous. **Intensive blood-glucose control with sulphonylureas or insulin compared with conventional treatment and risk of complications in patients with type 2 diabetes (UKPDS 33). United Kingdom Prospective Diabetes Study Group.** *Lancet* 1998, **352**:837–853.

25. Christensen CK, Krusell LR, Mogensen CE. **Increased blood pressure in diabetes: essential hypertension or diabetic nephropathy?** *Scand J Clin Lab Invest* 1987, **47**:363–370.

26. de Châtel R, Weidmann P, Flammer J *et al.* **Sodium, renin, aldosterone, catecholamines and blood pressure in diabetes mellitus.** *Kidney Int* 1977, **12**:412–421.

27. O'Hare JA, Ferriss JB, Brady D *et al.* **Exchangeable sodium and renin in hypertensive diabetic patients with and without nephropathy.** *Hypertension* 1985, **7** (suppl. 2):43–48.

28. DeFronzo RA. **The effect of insulin on renal sodium metabolism. A review with clinical implications.** *Diabetologia* 1981, **21**:165–171.

29. Hallab M, Bled F, Ebran JM. **Elevated serum angiotensin converting enzyme activity in type 1, insulin dependent diabetic subjects with persistent microalbuminuria.** *Acta Diabetol* 1992, **29**:82–85.

30. Drury PL, Smith GM, Ferris JB. **Increased vasopressor responsiveness to angiotensin II in type 1 (insulin-dependent) diabetic patients without nephropathy.** *Diabetologia* 1984, **27**:174–179.

31. Makarious M, Pawlak M, Campbell LV *et al.* **The platelet angiotensin II receptor in type I diabetes: studies in patients with and without nephropathy.** *Eur J Clin Invest* 1993, **23**:517–521.

32. Hostetter TH, Rennke HG, Brenner BM. **The case for intrarenal hypertension in the initiation and progression of diabetic and other glomerulopathies.** *Am J Med* 1982, **72**:375–380.

33. Zatz R, Brenner BM. **Pathogenesis of diabetic microangiopathy: the haemodynamic view.** *Am J Med* 1986, **80**:443–453.

34. Mogensen CE, Christensen CK. **Predicting diabetic nephropathy in insulin-dependent patients.** *N Engl J Med* 1984, **311**:89–93.

35. Makino H, Ikeda S, Haramoto T *et al.* **Heparan sulfate proteoglycans are lost in patients with diabetic nephropathy.** *Nephron* 1992, **61**:415–421.

36. Steffes MW, Brown DM, Mauer SM. **Diabetic glomerulopathy following unilateral nephrectomy in the rat.** *Diabetes* 1978, **27**:35–41.

37. Zatz R, Dunn BR, Meyer TW *et al.* **Prevention of diabetic glomerulopathy in pharmacological amelioration of glomerular capillary hypertension.** *J Clin Invest* 1986, **77**:1925–1930.

38. Christensen CK, Mogensen CE. **Effect of antihypertensive treatment on the progression of incipient diabetic nephropathy.** *Hypertension* 1985, **7** (suppl. 2): 109–113.

39. Agardh CD, Garcia-Puig J, Charbonnel B *et al.* **Greater reduction of urinary albumin excretion in hypertensive type II diabetic patients with incipient nephropathy by lisinopril than by nifedipine.** *J Hum Hyperten* 1996, **10**:185–192.

40. Anonymous. **Comparison between perindopril and nifedipine in hypertensive and normotensive diabetic patients with microalbuminuria. Melbourne Diabetic Nephropathy Study Group.** *Br Med J* 1991, **302**:210–216.

41. Hallab M, Gallois Y, Chatellier G *et al.* **Comparison of the reduction in microalbuminuria by enalapril and hydrochlorothiazide in normotensive patients with insulin dependent diabetes.** *Br Med J* 1993, **306**:175–182.

42. Mathiesen ER, Hommel E, Giese J *et al.* **Efficacy of captopril in postponing nephropathy in normotensive insulin dependent diabetic patients with microalbuminuria.** *Br Med J* 1991, **303**:81–87.

43. Marre M, Chatellier G, Leblanc H *et al.* **Prevention of diabetic nephropathy with enalapril in normotensive diabetics with microalbuminuria.** *Br Med J* 1988, **297**:1092–1095.

44. Anonymous. **Tight blood pressure control and risk of macrovascular and microvascular complications in type 2 diabetes: UKPDS 38. UK Prospective Diabetes Study Group.** *Br Med J* 1998, **317**:703–713.

45. Mogensen CE. **Progression of nephropathy in long-term diabetics with proteinuria and effect of initial antihypertensive treatment.** *Scand J Clin Lab Invest* 1976, **36**:383–388.

46. Parving HH, Andersen AR, Smidt UM *et al.* **Early aggressive antihypertensive treatment reduces rate of decline in kidney function in diabetic nephropathy.** *Lancet* 1983, **1**:1175–1179.

47. Lewis EJ, Hunsicker LG, Bain RP *et al.* **The effect of angiotensin-converting-enzyme inhibition on diabetic nephropathy. The Collaborative Study Group.** *N Engl J Med* 1993, **329**:1456–1462.

48. Lewis JB, Berl T, Bain RP *et al.* **Effects of intensive blood pressure control on the course of type 1 diabetic nephropathy. Collaborative Study Group.** *Am J Kidney Dis* 1999, **34**:809–817.

49. Ritz E, Strumpf C, Katz F *et al.* **Hypertension and cardiovascular risk factors in hemodialyzed diabetic patients.** *Hypertension* 1985, **7** (suppl. 2):118–124.

50. Friedman EA, Chou LM, Beyer M *et al.* **Adverse impact of hypertension on diabetic recipients of transplanted kidneys.** *Hypertension* 1985, **7** (suppl. 2):131–134.

51. Connell FA, Vadheim C, Emanuel I. **Diabetes and pregnancy: a population-based study of incidence, referral for care, and perinatal mortality.** *Am J Obstet Gynecol* 1985, **151**:598–603.

52. Anonymous. **Are ACE inhibitors safe in pregnancy?** *Lancet* 1989, **2**: 482–483.

53. Ramsay LE, Williams B, Johnston GD *et al.* **British Hypertension Society guidelines for hypertension management 1999: summary.** *Br Med J* 1999, **319**:630–635.

54. Nielsen FS, Rossing P, Gall MA *et al.* **Impact of lisinopril and atenolol on kidney function in hypertensive NIDDM subjects with diabetic nephropathy.** *Diabetes* 1994, **43**:1108–1113.

55. Elving LD, Wetzels JF, van Lier HJ *et al.* **Captopril and atenolol are equally effective in retarding progression of diabetic nephropathy. Results of a 2-year prospective, randomized study.** *Diabetologia* 1994, **37**:604–609.

56. Bakris GL, Barnhill BW, Sadler R. **Treatment of arterial hypertension in diabetic humans: importance of therapeutic selection.** *Kidney Int* 1992, **41**:912–919.

57. Davis JO. **What signals the kidney to release renin?** *Circ Res* 1971, **28**:301–306.

58. Parving HH, Hommel E, Smidt UM. **Protection of kidney function and decrease in albuminuria by captopril in insulin dependent diabetics with nephropathy.** *Br Med J* 1988, **297**:1086–1091.

59. Parving HH, Hommel E, Damkjaer Nielsen M *et al.* **Effect of captopril on blood pressure and kidney function in normotensive insulin dependent diabetics with nephropathy.** *Br Med J* 1989, **299**:533–536.

60. Björck S, Mulec H, Johnsen SA *et al.* **Renal protective effect of enalapril in diabetic nephropathy.** *Br Med J* 1992, **304**:339–343.

Pharmacology of antihypertensive drugs

Management of any chronic condition should avoid therapeutic agents that, while improving one risk factor, might have a deleterious effect on others. This is particularly true for the complex of the chronic cardiovascular risk factor syndrome (*see* Chapter 1). Hypertension is undoubtedly a major risk factor for both large and small vessel disease in patients with diabetes and adequate management is essential. Such management is made difficult because some of the drugs used may adversely affect glucose and lipid homeostasis, insulin sensitivity or interfere with metabolic and haemodynamic responses to hyperglycaemia and hypoglycaemia. In addition, patients with diabetes and complications such as autonomic neuropathy, peripheral vascular disease and renal disease may not be able to tolerate some of the antihypertensive drugs.

Blood pressure control in the diabetic patient with hypertension

Approaches to the general management of the diabetic patient with hypertension are considered in Chapter 6. Management includes dietary manipulation, correction of obesity, cessation of cigarette smoking, restriction of alcohol intake and often the use of pharmacological agents.

The ideal drug for the diabetic patient with hypertension should:

* lower blood pressure effectively;
* not impair glucose tolerance or interact with hypoglycaemics, or impair the patient's ability to recognise or respond to hyperglycaemia or to hypoglycaemia;
* not cause postural hypotension, impair limb blood flow, raise risk of impotence, or decrease renal function; and
* reduce susceptibility to ischaemic heart disease.

Major classes of antihypertensive drugs

Thiazide diuretics

These drugs are still commonly used as they are effective, inexpensive and can be given once daily.

They have, however, a number of possible adverse effects, and show a dose plateau above which enhanced blood pressure reduction is rare and adverse metabolic effects increase. Thiazides may be associated with several adverse metabolic effects, including deterioration in glycaemic control and precipitation of diabetes in those with impaired glucose tolerance and even in those without diabetes [1–3]. The reason for this is unknown but may relate to hypokalaemia [2]. Thiazides may also have a direct effect on the beta-cells of the pancreas, where they block insulin release [4], an effect that may worsen when thiazides are given in combination with a beta-blocker [5].

Thiazides have been shown to have adverse effects on the lipid profile, increasing total cholesterol, LDL-cholesterol and VLDL-cholesterol, with an overall increase in total triglycerides [6–8]. The mechanism of this effect is unknown, but may involve induction of insulin resistance with elevated plasma levels of both glucose and insulin [9,10]. Certainly, thiazides may be associated with increased insulin resistance, which may result in accelerated lipolysis and elevated circulating free fatty acids. In the presence of increased portal insulin levels, hepatic conversion of free fatty acids to triglycerides is accelerated.

Despite the above, it must be emphasised that many of these studies were carried out with doses of diuretic towards the higher range of that recommended; low-dose thiazides, which are just as effective in lowering blood pressure, are less likely to have such deleterious effects. It is generally accepted, however, that thiazides aggravate diabetic dyslipidaemia [11,12].

Other problems include impotence [13], particularly relevant in a condition such as diabetes where erectile impotence may occur in as many as 50% of patients. Thiazides, however, rarely cause postural hypotension and are unlikely to worsen peripheral vascular disease or renal function.

The above side effects must be weighed against the fact that the incidence of stroke and heart failure is lowered when severe and moderate hypertension are controlled with thiazides [14,15], and the incidence of stroke may be reduced by treating even mild hypertension [16]. The effects on CHD morbidity have been less consistent, with various studies showing, variously, no difference [17,18], deterioration [19,20], definite improvement [21–23] and a trend towards improvement [15,16,24]. One study also suggested an association between diuretic-induced hypokalaemia and cardiac arrhythmias [25], although this has been challenged [26].

Conclusion

Thiazides are recommended as first-line agents in patients without diabetes. Some authorities have not recommended their use as first-line agents in patients with diabetes because of adverse metabolic effects and precipitation of impotence. Use of low-dose diuretics is less likely to cause such problems and there is now evidence that shows reductions in cardiovascular disease and heart failure with these agents.

Beta-blockers

These drugs reduce cardiac output, heart rate and renal blood flow, and increase peripheral resistance. They are commonly used for the treatment of hypertension and are often effective and inexpensive: some may also be given in a once daily dosage. The use of beta-blockers in patients with diabetes, however, remains controversial. Certainly, cardioprotection and antianginal effects, the main advantages of beta-blockers, are often required in diabetic patients with hypertension. Beta-blockers are less likely to cause orthostatic hypotension compared with diuretics and possibly less erectile impotence, although this remains a problem.

There are, however, potential side effects, including adverse effects on glucose homeostasis. Stimulation of beta-adrenoceptors increases insulin release, immobilizes glucose from the liver, and produces the tachycardia and blood pressure changes associated with hypoglycaemia. Beta-blockade opposes these actions: most of these are $beta_2$-selective responses, so the more selective beta-blockers should have less effect [27].

Beta-blockade is associated with a high peak plasma glucose concentration in patients with and without diabetes [27,28], although this is less marked with a $beta_1$-selective blocker [27,29]. $Beta_2$-blockade may prolong hypoglycaemia by inhibiting glycogenolysis in muscles and lipolysis in adipose tissue, thus reducing the substrates available for gluconeo-

genesis and ketogenesis [30–34]. Perception of symptoms of hypoglycaemia may be impaired or altered by non-selective beta-blockers [30–32]. These problems have been reported to be rare, however, in prospective short-term [35] and long-term [36,37] trials in patients with type 1 or type 2 diabetes. Several studies have also demonstrated that recovery from insulin-induced hypoglycaemia is impaired by non-selective beta-blockade, although this happens to a lesser degree with cardioselective drugs [38]. Therefore, if beta-blockers are to be used, cardioselective agents are the preferred type.

Both selective and non-selective drugs may increase triglycerides and lower HDL-cholesterol, but whether these adverse effects are long term remains controversial [39]. Other problems include deterioration in peripheral vascular disease, as beta-blockers increase peripheral vascular resistance, promoting intermittent claudication and reduced limb perfusion.

Evidence suggests that beta-blockers may be cardioprotective. Beneficial effects of long-term beta-blockade following acute myocardial infarction are well-documented and are probably due, at least in part, to reduction in death from ventricular tachyarrhythmia [40–42]. In addition, the recently published hypertension arm of the UKPDS trial showed clear benefit from the point of view of tight blood pressure control in reducing cardiovascular risk and mortality in patients with type 2 diabetes, irrespective of whether an ACE inhibitor or a beta-blocker was used (see Chapter 5).

Conclusion

Although beta-blockers are often effective in lowering blood pressure and may have cardioprotective effects, their adverse metabolic effects may make the management of diabetes more difficult. Beta-blockers may, however, be particularly indicated in a person with type 2 diabetes who has hypertension and coincident angina. If a beta-blocker is to be used, a beta-selective drug is preferable.

Calcium antagonists

There are two groups of calcium antagonists, the dihydropyridines and the non-dihydropyridines. The non-dihydropyridines have been developed more recently and have a longer elimination half-life. These drugs provide 24-hour activity with a single daily dose and have fewer side effects. Not only do these drugs lower blood pressure but they have the added advantage of antianginal, cardioprotective and antiarrhythmic properties (Figure 4.1). In contrast to diuretics, they usually preserve cerebral and renal blood flow. Data from animal studies have suggested that they may prevent atherosclerosis; data from in-vitro studies suggest that they may inhibit platelet aggregation.

The antihypertensive action of calcium antagonists is based on their peripheral vasodilating properties, causing a direct decrease in total peripheral resistance [43]. Unfortunately, they produce side effects, usually minor and self-limiting, in a significant proportion of patients [44]. These include flushing, headaches and peripheral oedema.

Results from in-vitro animal studies show that these drugs might have a deleterious effect on glucose homeostasis. Reviews of studies, however, show no significant effect on glucose homeostasis in patients treated with calcium antagonists [45,46]. In addition, although data are limited, there appears to be no adverse effects on the lipid profile, as determined by measurements of total cholesterol, lipoprotein fractions and triglycerides [46,47]. Calcium antagonists also act as vasodilators, improving blood flow to the limbs, reducing the risk of impotence and perhaps providing benefit in peripheral vascular disease. Postural hypotension, particularly associated with autonomic neuropathy, is a problem for some patients with diabetes. This problem may be adversely affected by vasodilators, but not calcium antagonists. Most of the observed effects on the human kidney have been beneficial [48]. The overall effect may result from a series of different effects on systemic blood pressure, the intra-renal vasculature, renin release and tubular function. The natriuresis and diuresis caused by calcium antagonists help to counteract the tendency toward sodium and water retention observed in patients receiving other vasodilators. Renal disease does not substantially influence the pharmacokinetics of the available cal-

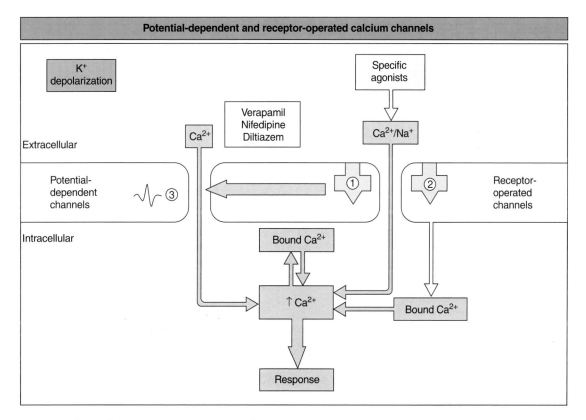

Figure 4.1. ① and ②, receptor-operated channels; ③, potential-dependent channel. Membrane depolarization activates ③, but can also be stimulated by agonists acting at ①. Receptor activation at ② can also lead to the release of intracellular calcium. ③ is sensitive to the action of verapamil, nifedipine and diltiazem. Adapted with the kind permission of Dr GD Johnston.

cium antagonists, which are eliminated by hepatic metabolism [48].

In coronary artery disease, calcium antagonists improve the coronary blood flow by dilating coronary arteries and possibly by reducing platelet stickiness. They should reduce the work that the heart is doing, by reducing afterload (through lowering peripheral vascular resistance) and by a direct effect on the myocardium. They may protect cells from ischaemia, which promotes a damaging influx of calcium, and exert an antiarrhythmic effect [49]. Regression of the structural changes of LVH has also been demonstrated in animals and humans [50].

Conclusion

Calcium antagonists can now be regarded as a first-line treatment in patients with diabetes and hypertension. They are relatively safe, with no clinically relevant metabolic side effects, but do have a high incidence of usually minor side effects. In addition, there is some evidence of cardioprotective properties, with the potential to improve peripheral circulation and renal function. There are now significant trial data, involving subgroup analysis of

patients with diabetes in the recently published Systolic Hypertension in Europe study (SYST-Eur), which shows that treatment of systolic hypertension in elderly patients with diabetes is beneficial in reducing total mortality, cardiovascular mortality and cardiovascular end points, as compared with placebo. Calcium antagonist therapy was the active intervention in this study (*see* Chapter 5).

Angiotensin-converting enzyme inhibitors

The RAS has an important role in the control of blood pressure, fluids and electrolytes (Figure 4.2). Angiotensin II is a powerful vasoconstrictor and mediator of adrenocortical aldosterone secretion. It also appears to have an effect on the sympathetic nervous system, enhancing the release of noradrenaline from nerve endings and inhibiting presynaptic uptake. Inhibition of the RAS was the objective in the development of the ACE inhibitors [51]. The antihypertensive action of these agents may, in part, be caused by a reduction of sympathetic tone, which is mediated by withdrawal of the facilitative action of angiotensin II on sympathetic neurotransmission. Other effects of angiotensin II on parasympathetic

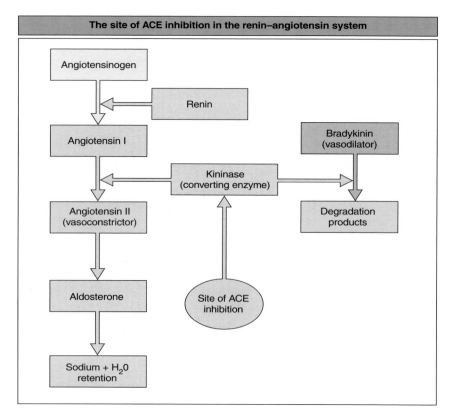

The site of ACE inhibition in the renin–angiotensin system

Figure 4.2. ACE, angiotensin-converting enzyme.

circulatory control, and perhaps on resistance vessel structure, may be important.

ACE inhibitors lower blood pressure by decreasing elevated systemic vascular resistance, but do not produce reflex sympathetic activation or alter myocardial conductivity. They enhance perfusion of vital organs, reverse cardiac hypertrophy and have beneficial effects in patients with congestive heart failure, improving the clinical state and prolonging life. Both preload and afterload are decreased and, because there is no risk of reflex tachycardia, cardiac oxygen demands are decreased. Potential problems with ACE inhibitors include renal impairment and bone marrow suppression, which may be dose-related. A range of ACE inhibitors are now available. ACE inhibitors are eliminated by the kidneys and, as both age and cardiovascular disease are factors that impair renal function, there is an increased potential for adverse reactions in patients with renal impairment [52], therefore, these agents should be used with caution.

ACE inhibitors have been associated with hypotension after the first dose, most often seen in those receiving diuretics. If possible, it is wise to stop or reduce diuretics one or two days before commencing ACE inhibitor therapy. In practice, provided that the patient is started on a low dose of ACE inhibitor, first-dose hypotension is now rare. A characteristic cough with a tickling sensation in the throat, and sometimes nasal stuffiness and wheezing, has also been associated with these drugs. The problem tends to diminish with time and may be related to inhibition of enzymes that break down bradykinin.

There are several potential advantages of using ACE inhibitors in the diabetic patient with hypertension.

Glucose homeostasis

The effect of ACE inhibitors on glucose metabolism has been evaluated in several controlled studies [53–55]. They were found to be safe and effective in treating hypertension. Glucose metabolism was not affected and, indeed, some studies showed improvement in glycaemia [56]. No patients required changes in the doses of insulin or oral hypoglycaemic drugs, although one recent report, based on hospital reporting statistics, has suggested an increased susceptibility to hypoglycaemia in both sulphonylurea-treated and insulin-treated patients with diabetes [57]. All drugs in this class tend to reduce insulin resistance and, therefore, increase insulin sensitivity [46].

Serum lipids

No deleterious effects on the lipid profile have been demonstrated in patients with diabetes treated with ACE inhibitors. Indeed, several studies have suggested an improvement in lipids, including an increase in the HDL-cholesterol:total cholesterol ratio in hypertensive patients with or without dyslipidaemia (likely to be beneficial) [58–60].

Complications of diabetes

Treatment of hypertension is important in reducing the rate of decline of renal function in overt diabetic nephropathy. This is particularly the case with ACE inhibitors [46] (*see* Chapter 3), perhaps because of intra-renal effects on the renal microcirculation over and above their systemic blood pressure lowering effects. Reports of improvement in renal function, even in patients with microalbuminuria who are normotensive, suggest that this improvement may be specifically related to ACE inhibition rather than to the general effects of systemic blood pressure.

In addition to ACE inhibition slowing decline in renal function in overt nephropathy, a recent large study has demonstrated not only a significant slowing of progression to ESRF, but also reduced mortality, in patients with overt nephropathy and diabetes [61]. A recent study has demonstrated that a combination of ACE inhibition and intensive blood pressure control can result in regression of clinical signs of diabetic nephropathy [62]. There is also evidence that patients with incipient nephropathy, even those who are normotensive, may be prevented from progressing to overt nephropathy by using ACE inhibitors (*see* Chapter 3). These studies have, however, tended to be performed on small numbers of patients for a short duration. Long-term studies have shown that ACE inhibition not only delays, but also may prevent, the establishment of diabetic glomerulopathy [63].

ACE inhibitors should be used with caution in patients with severe renal impairment (creatinine >200 mmol/l), as renal impairment may be worsened. Caution should also be exercised in elderly patients who may have atherosclerotic-related renal artery stenosis, as again renal function may deteriorate rapidly. Serum creatinine should be measured immediately before and a few days after starting ACE inhibitor therapy.

ACE inhibitors do not cause impotence, and any effect on peripheral vascular disease is likely to be beneficial.

Ischaemic heart disease

ACE inhibitors, in combination with diuretics, are now well-established as a suitable treatment for heart failure. Evidence of benefit after myocardial infarction is accruing, including positive effects on mortality both in heart failure and after myocardial infarction. In hypertensive patients without diabetes, ACE inhibition is associated with regression of structural changes in hypertrophied myocardium [64], and this may also be the case in those with diabetes. Early treatment with an ACE inhibitor in patients with diabetes and acute myocardial infarction is associated with a decreased six-week mortality [65].

The Heart Outcomes Prevention Evaluation (HOPE) study reported the efficacy of the ACE inhibitor, ramipril, on the incidence of myocardial infarction, stroke or cardiovascular death in people at high risk of cardiovascular disease [66]. The study was multi-centre, international and randomized, with over 9,500 patients, 3,500 of whom had diabetes, and a planned follow up of five years. All patients were over 55 years of age, and patients without diabetes had a history of previous cardiovascular disease. Those with diabetes had either a history of previous cardiovascular disease, or one other cardiovascular risk factor, such as total cholesterol greater than 5.2 mmol/l, HDL-cholesterol less than 0.9 mmol/l, treated hypertension or untreated blood pressure greater than 160/90 mmHg, smoking or microalbuminuria. Of the 3,500 patients with diabetes, 56% had hypertension.

In the groups with and without diabetes there was a clear split in survival curves in favour of those on ACE inhibitor treatment, such that the trial was discontinued early, at 4.5 years. There was a highly significant reduction in mortality in the whole group (22%) and in the subgroup with diabetes (24%), as compared with placebo. In addition, there were significant reductions in myocardial infarction (22%), in stroke (33%; $P<0.01$), in transient ischaemic attack (26%) and in cardiovascular death (37%). Benefit was apparent between six and eight months after randomization, and was seen despite the fact that both the control and active groups could have any other therapies prescribed. Overall, ACE inhibitor treatment was associated with reduced incidence of cardiovascular death, of stroke and of myocardial

infarction in patients at high risk of cardiovascular disease, including patients with diabetes. The additional reduction in systolic blood pressure (3 mmHg) and diastolic blood pressure (2 mmHg) in the ACE inhibitor-treated group would, based on the results of other trials, translate to a 13% reduction in stroke and 5% reduction in myocardial infarction. The HOPE study, however, demonstrated a 33% reduction in stroke and a 22% reduction in myocardial infarction, suggesting a benefit of ACE inhibitors over and above their blood pressure lowering effect.

In addition, there is now good evidence for renal protection using ACE inhibitors (*see* Chapter 3) and emerging evidence from the Eurodiab Controlled Trial of Lisinopril in Insulin-Dependent Diabetes (EUCLID) study (*see* Chapter 5) that they may protect against progression of diabetic retinopathy [67].

Conclusion

ACE inhibitors enjoy a high level of patient acceptability as they have no demonstrable psychological or physiological effects. They may also have specific beneficial effects on diabetic nephropathy and retinopathy and in the management of heart failure and after myocardial infarction. Recent data from the HOPE study suggest that ACE inhibitors may also be of great benefit in patients with diabetes who have at least one other cardiovascular risk factor or who have had a previous cardiovascular event, with regard to reduction in overall mortality, cardiovascular mortality and cardiovascular end points. Cardiovascular protection may occur, at least in part, irrespective of their blood pressure lowering effects. Overall, they are effective anti-hypertensive agents that do not cause adverse metabolic effects (Table 4.1).

Angiotensin II antagonists (angiotensin type 1 receptor blockers)

This is a relatively new class of agent that specifically block the effect of angiotensin II at the (type 1) receptor site [68]. Their efficacy in blood pressure lowering is comparable with ACE inhibitors and other antihypertensive agents, with an excellent metabolic profile. They also do not cause the chronic cough, which may sometimes be associated with ACE inhibitors.

They have been shown to be as effective as ACE inhibitors in delaying progression of renal injury in animal models [69]. Small clinical studies have also demonstrated improvement in markers of 'renal pro-

Effects of antihypertensive drugs on patients with diabetes						
	Thiazides	Beta-blockers	Alpha-blockers	Calcium antagonists	ACE inhibitors	Angiotensin II antagonists
Glucose	↑	↑	N	N	N	N
Lipids	↑	↑#	N	N	N	N
Electrolytes	*	N	N	N	N	N
Insulin resistance	↑	↑	↓#	N	↓#	↓#
Complications of diabetes						
Cardiovascular	+	+	N/A	+	+	N/A
Microvascular	N/A	+	N/A	N/A	+	N/A
Impotence	–	–	N	N	N	N

Table 4.1. ACE, angiotensin-converting enzyme; ↑, deterioration; ↓, improvement; #, not yet clinically established; N, neutral; *, electrolyte disturbance can occur; +, protection; –, worsening; N/A, no data available. There is evidence of renal protection with angiotensin II antagonists in animal models of the disease and in short-term human trials that used surrogate markers; results from trials underway are awaited.

tection' compared with calcium antagonists, and equal blood pressure lowering effects [70]. There are several trials underway using a range of angiotensin II antagonists in patients with diabetes to determine whether or not they are as effective as ACE inhibitors in renal protection and retinopathy in humans.

A recent report has also shown equal blood pressure lowering in patients with type 2 diabetes using either the ACE inhibitor, lisinopril, or the angiotensin II antagonist, candesartan cilexetil. The combination of these two agents, however, produces a further significant fall in blood pressure, with a nonsignificant tendency to further reduction of the urinary albumin:creatinine ratio. This suggests that combining these two drugs, both of which effect the RAS (in different ways), is likely to produce clinical benefit, although further work in this area is required [71].

In addition, mortality and morbidity studies on several thousand patients with hypertension, heart failure, diabetes with renal impairment and after myocardial infarction are currently ongoing using various angiotensin II antagonists. Although these agents look interesting, they need further evaluation in the management of patients with hypertension and diabetes. It is certainly possible that, with time, they too may become first-line agents.

Other drugs

A range of other drugs is also available. Many of these drugs are rarely used in hypertensive practice, but some of the newer drugs on the market may be of benefit in patients with diabetes, although they require further evaluation. These include the specific alpha-blockers, which decrease peripheral vascular resistance and cause venous dilatation, thus decreasing venous return to the right side of the heart. This may be an advantage over direct vasodilatation in patients with ischaemic heart disease, as cardiac output is not significantly increased. Older drugs, such as prazosin, may show severe initial first-dose hypotension and some patients with diabetes have persistent orthostatic hypotension with this drug. The new alpha-blockers are, however, reported to be better tolerated, with no significant deleterious metabolic side effects [72,73]. With further evaluation they may become established first-line agents.

An agent that is difficult to classify, but which may be useful in patients with diabetes and hypertension, is indapamide. This reduces the increased vascular sensitivity to circulating pressor amines and vasodilatation. It also appears to have an initial diuretic effect in some patients. There is a chemical relationship between indapamide and thiazide diuretics, but no evidence that indapamide precipitates diabetes or causes problems in patients who already have diabetes at the time of starting treatment [74].

A recently introduced, centrally acting antihypertensive agent, moxonidine, which is a selective imidazoline receptor agonist, also looks to be of interest. Preliminary data suggest metabolic neutrality [75] and reduced side effects compared with the older, centrally acting agents, such as clonidine and methyldopa. Further information is awaited.

Summary

Suggested management regimens are reviewed in Chapter 6. Reviewing the known pharmacological profiles of the various classes of antihypertensives suggests that both calcium antagonists and, in particular, ACE inhibitors should now be considered as first-line treatments for hypertension in patients with diabetes. New angiotensin II antagonists may be of similar use, but further information, particularly in patients with diabetes, is awaited.

Beta-blockers are acceptable alternatives, particularly if there are other indications such as angina or after myocardial infarction. Specific alpha-blockers may also be useful but again hard end point data are awaited. Thiazide diuretics should be avoided, if possible, as first-line agents, but can be useful in combination with other antihypertensives, particularly ACE inhibitors. If thiazides are used, they should be administered at low doses, as antihypertensive efficacy is equivalent to higher doses but with a significantly reduced risk of deleterious side effects. If single drug treatment fails to achieve adequate control, which is common, then combination therapy with different classes of antihypertensive agents should be used.

References

1. Murphy MB, Lewis PJ, Kohner E *et al.* **Glucose intolerance in hypertensive patients treated with diuretics; a fourteen-year follow-up.** *Lancet* 1982, 2:1293–1295.

2. Amery A, Berthoux P, Bulpitt C *et al.* **Glucose intolerance during diuretic therapy. Results of trial by the European Working Party on Hypertension in the Elderly.** *Lancet* 1978, 1:681–683.

3. Lewis PJ, Kohner EM, Petrie A *et al.* **Deterioration of glucose tolerance in hypertensive patients on prolonged diuretic treatment.** *Lancet* 1976, 1:564–566.

4. Strathers AD, Murphy MB, Dollery CT. **Glucose tolerance during antihypertensive therapy in patients with diabetes mellitus.** *Hypertension* 1975, 7 (suppl. 2):95–101.

5. Dornhorst A, Powell SH, Pensky J. **Aggravation by propranolol of hyperglycaemic effect of hydrochlorothiazide in type II diabetics without alteration of insulin secretion.** *Lancet* 1985, 1:123–126.

6. Schoenfeld MR, Goldberger E. **Hypercholesterolaemia induced by thiazides: a pilot study.** *Curr Ther Res* 1964, 6:180–184.

7. Kannel WB, Castelli WP. **Is the serum total cholesterol an anachronism?** *Lancet* 1979, 2:950–951.

8. Ames RP. **Coronary heart disease and the treatment of hypertension: impact of diuretics on serum lipids and glucose.** *J Cardiovasc Pharmacol* 1984, 6 (suppl. 3):S466–S473.

9. Ames RP. **The effects of antihypertensive drugs on serum lipids and lipoproteins. I. Diuretics.** *Drugs* 1986, 32:260–278.

10. Ames RP, Hill P. **Antihypertensive therapy and the risk of coronary heart disease.** *J Cardiovasc Pharmacol* 1982, 4 (suppl. 2):S206–S212.

11. Ferrari P, Rosman J, Weidmann P. **Antihypertensive agents, serum lipoprotein and glucose metabolism.** *Am J Cardiol* 1991, 67:26B–35B.

12. Weidmann P, de Courten M, Ferrari P. **Effect of diuretics on plasma lipid profile.** *Eur Heart J* 1992, 13 (suppl. G):61–67.

13. Anonymous. **Adverse reactions to bendrofluazide and propranolol for the treatment of mild hypertension. Report of Medical Research Council Working Party on Mild to Moderate Hypertension.** *Lancet* 1981, 2:539–543.

14. Anonymous. **Effects of treatment on morbidity in hypertension. Results in patients with diastolic blood pressure averaging 115 through 129 mm Hg.** *JAMA* 1967, 202:1028–1034.

15. Anonymous. **Effects of treatment on morbidity in hypertension. II. Results in patients with diastolic blood pressure averaging 90 through 114 mm Hg.** *JAMA* 1970, 213:1143–1152.

16. Anonymous. **MRC trial of treatment of mild hypertension: principal results. Medical Research Council Working Party.** *Br Med J (Clin Res Ed)* 1985, 291:97–104.

17. Helgeland A. **Treatment of mild hypertension: a five year controlled drug trial. The Oslo Study.** *Am J Med* 1980, 69:725–732.

18. Anonymous. **Multiple risk factor intervention trial. Risk factor changes and mortality results. Multiple Risk Factor Intervention Trial Research Group.** *JAMA* 1982, 248:1465–1477.

19. Jones JV, Dunn FG, Fife R *et al.* **Benzothiadiazine diuretics and death from myocardial infarction in hypertension.** *Clin Sci Mol Med Suppl* 1978, 4:315s–317s.

20. Morgan TO, Adams WR, Hodgson M *et al.* **Failure of therapy to improve prognosis in elderly males with hypertension.** *Med J Aust* 1980, 2:27–31.

21. Anonymous. **Five-year findings of the hypertension detection and follow-up program. I. Reduction in mortality in persons with high blood pressure including mild hypertension. Hypertension Detection and Follow-up Program Cooperative Group.** *JAMA* 1979, 242:2562–2571.

22. Berglund G, Sannerstedt R, Andersson O *et al.* **Coronary heart disease after treatment of hypertension.** *Lancet* 1978, 1:1–5.

23. Amery A, Birkenhäger W, Brixko P et al. **Mortality and morbidity results from the European Working Party on High Blood Pressure in the Elderly trial.** Lancet 1985, 1:1349–1354.

24. Anonymous. **The Australian therapeutic trial in mild hypertension. Report by the Management Committee.** Lancet 1980, 1:1261–1267.

25. Holland OB, Nixon JV, Kuhnert L. **Diuretic-induced ventricular ectopic activity.** Am J Med 1981, **70**:762–768.

26. Papademetriou V. **Diuretics, hypokalemia and cardiac arrhythmias: a critical analysis.** Am Heart J 1986, **111**:1217–1224.

27. Kendall MJ. **Are selective beta-adrenoceptor blocking drugs an advantage?** J R Coll Physicians Lond 1981, **15**:33–40.

28. Pollare T, Lithell H, Selinus I et al. **Sensitivity to insulin during treatment with atenolol and metoprolol: a randomised, double blind study of effects on carbohydrate and lipoprotein metabolism in hypertensive patients.** Br Med J 1989, **298**:1152–1157.

29. Wright AD, Barber SG, Kendall MJ et al. **Beta-adrenoceptor-blocking drugs and blood sugar control in diabetes mellitus.** Br Med J 1979, 1:159–161.

30. Waal-Manning HJ. **Can beta-blockers be used in diabetic patients?** Drugs 1979, **17**;157–160.

31. Christlieb AR, Maki PC. **The effect of beta-blocker therapy on glucose and lipid metabolism.** Prim Cardiol 1980, **(suppl.)**:47–54.

32. Ostman J. **Beta-adrenergic blockade and diabetes mellitus. A review.** Acta Med Scand Suppl 1983, **672**:69–77.

33. Deacon SP, Karunanayake A, Barnett D. **Acebutolol, atenolol and propranolol and metabolic responses to acute hypoglycaemia in diabetics.** Br Med J 1977, **2**:1255–1257.

34. Lager I, Blohmé G, Smith U. **Effect of cardioselective and non-selective beta-blockade on the hypoglycaemic response in insulin dependent diabetics.** Lancet 1979, 1:458–462.

35. Ryan JR, LaCorte W, Jain A et al. **Hypertension in hypoglycaemic diabetics treated with beta-adrenergic antagonists.** Hypertension 1985, **7**:443–446.

36. Barnett AH, Leslie D, Watkins PJ. **Can insulin-treated diabetics be given beta-adrenergic blocking drugs?** Br Med J 1980, **280**:976–978.

37. Kølendorf K, Bonnevie-Neilsen V, Broch-Møller B. **A trial of metoprolol in hypertensive insulin-dependent diabetic patients.** Acta Med Scand 1982, **211**:175–178.

38. Deacon SP, Barnett D. **Comparison of atenolol and propranolol during insulin-inducted hypoglycaemia.** Br Med J 1976, **2**:272–273.

39. Ames RP. **The effect of antihypertensive drugs on serum lipids and lipoproteins. II. Non-diuretic drugs.** Drugs 1986, **32**:335–357.

40. Hearse DJ, Yellon DM, Downey JM. **Can beta blockers limit myocardial infarct size?** Eur Heart J 1986, **7**:925–930.

41. Rydén L, Ariniego R, Arnman K et al. **A double-blind trial of metoprolol in acute myocardial infarction. Effects on ventricular tachyarrhythmias.** N Engl J Med 1983, **308**:614–618.

42. Yusuf S, Peto R, Lewis J et al. **Beta-blockade during and after myocardial infarction: an overview of the randomized trials.** Prog Cardiovasc Dis 1985, **27**:335–371.

43. Vanhoutte P. **Calcium-entry blockers, vascular smooth muscle and systemic hypertension [Abstract].** Am J Cardiol 1985, **55**:17B.

44. Gill JS, Zezulka AV, Beevers M et al. **An audit of nifedipine in a hypertension clinic.** J Clin Hosp Pharmacol 1986, **11**:107–116.

45. Trost BN, Weidmann P. **Effects of calcium antagonists on glucose homeostasis and serum lipids in non-diabetic and diabetic subjects: a review.** J Hypertens Suppl 1987, **5**:S81–S104.

46. Maxwell SRB, Barnett AH. **The management of hypertension in the diabetic patient.** In Difficult Hypertension. Edited by MJ Kendall, NM Kaplan and RC Horton. London: Martin Dunitz, 1995;135–160.

47. Faergeman O, Meinertz H, Hansen JF. **Serum lipoproteins after treatment with verapamil for 6 months.** Acta Med Scand Suppl 1984, **681**:49–51.

48. Chellingsworth M, Kendall MJ. **Calcium antagonists and the kidney.** J Hum Hypertens 1987, 1:3–8.

49. Kendall MJ, Horton RC. **Are calcium antagonists cardioprotective?** J R Coll Physicians Lond 1985, **19**: 85–89.

50. Agabiti-Rosei E, Muiesan ML, Romanelli G et al. **Reversal of cardiac hypertrophy by long-term treatment with calcium antagonists in hypertensive patients.** J Cardiovasc Pharmacol 1988, **12** (suppl. 6):S75–S78.

51. Brown JJ, Casals-Stenzel J, Cumming AMM et al. **Angiotensin II, aldosterone and arterial pressure: a quantitative approach.** Hypertension 1979, 1:159–179.

52. Thomson AH, Kelly JG, Whiting B. **Lisinopril population pharmacokinetics in elderly and renal disease patients with hypertension.** Br J Clin Pharmacol 1989, **27**:57–65.

53. Sullivan PA, Kelleher M, Twomey M et al. **Effects of converting enzyme inhibition on blood pressure, plasma renin activity (PRA) and plasma aldosterone in hypertensive diabetics compared to patients with essential hypertension.** J Hypertens 1985, **3**:359–363.

54. Gambaro G, Morbiato F, Cicerello E et al. **Captopril in the treatment of hypertension in type I and type II diabetic patients.** J Hypertens Suppl 1985, **3**:S149–S151.

55. Matthews DM, Wathen CG, Bell D et al. **The effect of captopril on blood pressure and glucose tolerance in hypertensive non-insulin dependent diabetics.** Postgrad Med J 1986, **62** (suppl. 1):73–75.

56. Bergemann R, Wohler D, Weidmann P et al. **[Improved glucose regulation and microalbuminuria/proteinuria in diabetic patients treated with ACE inhibitors. A meta-analysis of published studies of 1985–1990.]** Schweiz Med Wochenschr 1992, **122**:1369–1376.

57. Herings RM, de Boer A, Stricker BH et al. **Hypoglycaemia associated with the use of inhibitors of**

angiotensin converting enzyme. *Lancet* 1995, **345**: 1195–1198.

58. Shionoiri H, Veda S, Gotch E *et al.* **Glucose and lipid metabolism during long term lisinopril therapy in hypertensive patients.** *J Cardiovasc Pharmacol* 1990, **16**:905–909.

59. Paolisso G, Gambardella A, Verza M *et al.* **ACE-inhibition improves insulin-sensitivity in aged insulin-resistant hypertensive patients.** *J Hum Hypertens* 1992, **6**:175–179.

60. Bak JF, Gerdes LU, Sørensen NS *et al.* **Effects of perindopril on insulin sensitivity and plasma lipid profile in hypertensive non-insulin-dependent diabetic patients.** *Am J Med* 1992, **92** (suppl. 4B):69S–72S.

61. Lewis EJ, Hunsicker LG, Bain RP *et al.* **The effect of angiotensin-converting enzyme inhibition on diabetic nephropathy. The Collaborative Study Group.** *N Engl J Med* 1993, **329**:1456–1462.

62. Lewis JB, Berl T, Bain RP *et al.* **Effects of intensive blood pressure control on the course of type I diabetic nephropathy. Collaborative Study Group.** *Am J Kidney Dis* 1999, **34**:809–817.

63. Zatz R, Dunn AR, Meyer TW *et al.* **Prevention of diabetic glomerulopathy by pharmacological amelioration of glomerular capillary hypertension.** *J Clin Invest* 1986, **77**:1925–1930.

64. Cruickshank JM, Lewis J, Moore V *et al.* **Reversibility of left ventricular hypertrophy by differing types of antihypertensive therapy.** *J Hum Hypertens* 1992, **6**:85–90.

65. Zuanetti G, Latini R, Maggioni AP *et al.* **Effect of the ACE inhibitor lisinopril on mortality in diabetic patients with acute myocardial infarction: data from the GISSI-3 study.** *Circulation* 1997, **96**:4239–4245.

66. Anonymous. **Effects of ramipril on cardiovascular and microvascular outcomes in people with diabetes mellitus: results of the HOPE study and MICRO-HOPE substudy. Heart Outcomes Prevention Evaluation Study Investigators.** *Lancet* 2000, **355**:253–259.

67. Chaturvedi N, Sjolie AK, Stephenson JM *et al.* **Effect of lisinopril on progression of retinopathy in people with type 1 diabetes. The EUCLID Study Group. EURODIAB Controlled Trial of Lisinopril in Insulin-Dependent Diabetes Mellitus.** *Lancet* 1998, **351**:28–31.

68. Timmermans PBMWM. **The discovery and physiological effects of a new class of highly specific angiotensin-II receptor antagonists.** In *Hypertension Pathophysiology, Diagnosis and Management.* Edited by JH Laragh and BM Brenner. New York: Raven Press, 1990;2351–2360.

69. Mackenzie HS, Provoost AP, Troy JL *et al.* **Antihypertensive and renal protective effects of irbesartan in fawn-hooded hypertensive rats.** *J Hypertens* 1996, **14** (suppl. 1):S42.

70. Pohl M, Cooper M, Ulrey J *et al.* **Safety and efficacy of irbesartan in hypertensive patients with type II diabetes and proteinuria.** *Am J Hypertens* 1997, **10**:105A.

71. Mogensen CE. **Intervention strategies for microalbuminuria: the role of angiotensin II antagonists, including dual blockade with ACE-I and a receptor blocker [Abstract].** Third International Symposium on Angiotensin II Antagonism, London, UK. 2000; A7.4.

72. Feher MD. **Doxazosin therapy in the treatment of diabetic hypertension.** *Am Heart J* 1991, **121**:1294–1301.

73. Weidmann P, de Courten M, Ferrari P. **Effect of diuretics on the plasma lipid profile.** *Eur Heart J* 1992, **13** (suppl. G):1–7.

74. Roux P, Courtois H. **Blood sugar regulation during treatment with indapamide in hypertensive diabetics [Abstract].** *Postgrad Med J* 1981, **57** (suppl. 12):70.

75. Krentz AJ, Evans AJ. **Selective imidazoline receptor agonists for metabolic syndrome.** *Lancet* 1998, **351**:152–153.

Benefit of hypertensive treatment in patients with diabetes: recent trials

Until recently, the benefit of treating hypertension in patients with diabetes was determined by extrapolation of data from large antihypertensive treatment trials in patients without diabetes. While this was a logical approach, recent data has demonstrated that the patient with diabetes poses special problems. These problems include:

- the potential for adverse effects of antihypertensive treatment on the other metabolic abnormalities in diabetes (eg, thiazides and dyslipidaemia);
- effects on microvascular disease; and
- concerns over the J-shaped hypothesis, which suggests that lowering blood pressure below a certain level may increase mortality.

Reports of increased morbidity and mortality in association with calcium antagonist treatment in patients without diabetes also caused considerable concern. This was based on analysis of trial data that showed a high incidence of coronary artery disease in patients treated with calcium antagonists compared with those treated with ACE inhibitors (eg, Appropriate Blood Pressure Control in Diabetes [ABCD], Flosequinan-ACE inhibitor Trial [FACET] and Multicenter Isradipine Diuretic Atherosclerosis Study [MIDAS]) [1].

A number of recently published, large hypertension trials have, however, included substantial numbers of patients with diabetes, allowing separate subgroup analysis to be conducted on diabetic patients with hypertension alone [1]. In two of these trials, it was the subgroup with diabetes that showed the most persuasive results for treatment of hypertension (HOT and Captopril Prevention Project [CAPPP], *see* below).

Effects of antihypertensive therapy on mortality and morbidity in diabetic patients with hypertension

Six large, randomized, prospective trials have confirmed the considerable benefit of antihypertensive treatment on cardiovascular outcome in patients with diabetes (Systolic Hypertension in the Elderly Program [SHEP], UKPDS, HOT, SYST-Eur, HOPE and CAPPP) [2–7]. These trials are summarized in Table 5.1.

Five hundred and eighty-three elderly patients with diabetes were included in the placebo-controlled SHEP study, where patients were allocated to receive treatment with chlorthalidone, with or without atenolol or reserpine [2]. The results showed a reduction in systolic blood pressure that was 9.8 mmHg lower than the control group and a reduction in the relative risk of myocardial infarction (46%). This is a reassuring finding in view of the potential adverse effects of beta-blockers and thiazides in patients with diabetes.

Within the factorial design of the UKPDS [3], a multicentre, randomized, controlled trial of tight blood pressure control versus less tight blood pressure control was undertaken. The mean difference between treatment groups in systolic blood pressure and diastolic blood pressure was 10 mmHg and 5 mmHg, respectively, in favour of the tightly controlled group. After nine-years follow up, reductions of 32% in diabetes-related deaths, 44% in strokes and 34% in combined macrovascular end points were seen. The study also confirmed the substantial benefit of hypertension treatment for microvascular end points (37% reduction, predominantly caused by the reduced risk of progression to retinopathy and retinal photocoagulation). This landmark study also demonstrated the cost-effectiveness of tight blood pressure control in type 2 diabetic patients with hypertension [8], and suggested a target blood pressure with therapy of 140 mmHg systolic and 85 mmHg diastolic. It also emphasised that, to achieve this target, at least 60% of patients required two or more different antihypertensive agents.

The impressive benefit with therapy and the target blood pressure suggested by the hypertension arm of the UKPDS have been reinforced by the large HOT study [4]. The HOT study included 1,501 diabetic patients with hypertension who were randomly allocated to three different diastolic blood pressure targets (<90, <85 and <80 mmHg). In addition, half of

Recent randomized, controlled trials of hypertension-related treatment in subjects with diabetes						
Trial	Patients (*n*)	Follow-up (years)	Treatment	Fall in blood pressure (mmHg)	Reduction in end points summary	Implication?
SHEP	583	5	Thiazide and beta-blocker	9.8/2.2	All cardiovascular disease events (46–66%)	Thiazides and beta-blockers effective
UKPDS	1,148	9	Captopril or atenolol	10/5	Strokes (44%), diabetes-related deaths (32%), microvascular end points (37%)	Target blood pressure achieved <140/85 mmHg; cost-effective; microvascular event reduction; no apparent difference between ACE inhibitors and beta-blockers
HOT	1,501	4	Calcium antagonist	29.9/24.3	Major cardiovascular events and total mortality (50%)	Target <140/85 mmHg; two or more agents commonly required; safety of calcium antagonists confirmed
SYST-Eur	492	2	Calcium antagonist	10.11/4.5	All major cardiovascular events (41–70%)	Calcium antagonists safe and effective; impressive reductions in mortality
CAPPP	552	6	Captopril versus beta-blocker or thiazide	Both 16/10	Captopril group reduced fatal and non-fatal MI by 34%	Suggests effectiveness of ACE inhibition
MICRO-HOPE	3,577	4.5	ACE inhibition in high-risk subjects	2.4/1.0*	Total mortality (−24%), MI (−22%), stroke (−33%), microvascular (−16%)	Benefit even in normotensive patients (42%); ACE inhibition safe and effective; treat those with microvascular disease (particularly early nephropathy)
EUCLID	530	2	ACE inhibition	3/2*	Progression of retinopathy	ACE inhibition may have a specific retinoprotective effect
STENO II	160	3.8	ACE inhibition; tight glycaemic and lipid control		Less progression to macroalbuminuria (27%) and retinopathy (45%)	Multifactorial intervention

Table 5.1. All the trials included patients with type 2 diabetes except the Eurodiab Controlled Trial of Lisinopril in Insulin-Dependent Diabetes (EUCLID), which included normotensive patients with type 1 diabetes. SHEP, Systolic Hypertension in the Elderly Program; UKPDS, UK Prospective Diabetes Study; HOT, Hypertension Optimal Treatment; SYST-Eur, Systolic Hypertension in Europe Study; CAPPP, Captopril Prevention Project; MICRO-HOPE, Microalbuminuria, Cardiovascular, and Renal Outcomes in the Heart Outcomes Prevention Evaluation; ACE, angiotensin-converting enzyme; MI, myocardial infarction. *many patients normotensive at entry.

the patients in each treatment group were randomly allocated to receive aspirin; the treatment used was a calcium antagonist. The study demonstrated that the group of diabetic patients with hypertension achieving a mean systolic blood pressure of 139.7 mmHg and mean diastolic blood pressure of 81.1 mmHg had half the number of cardiovascular events compared with the group with less tight control who were allocated to a target diastolic blood pressure of below 90 mmHg. Although the reduction of blood pressure below these levels was not associated with increased benefit, reassuringly it was also not associated with increased mortality (allaying fears based on the J-shaped curve hypothesis). The HOT study also provided the first evidence for the benefit of aspirin as a primary prevention therapy in diabetic patients with hypertension. This therapy further reduced cardiovascular events by 15%, but at the expense of more non-fatal bleeding events.

Evidence derived from the HOT study is, therefore, in agreement with the findings of the hypertension arm of the UKPDS with regard to target blood pressure, threshold for treatment and the number of patients requiring two or more agents to achieve tight blood pressure control. The HOT study also established the benefit of aspirin in primary prevention in diabetic patients with hypertension and allayed fears about the safety of the calcium antagonists.

A subgroup analysis of 492 diabetic patients with hypertension in the large SYST-Eur trial [5] has also confirmed the benefit of calcium antagonist therapy. The principal results of this subgroup analysis demonstrated that calcium antagonist-based therapy led to impressive reductions of 55% in total mortality, 76% in cardiovascular mortality and 73% in strokes, as compared with placebo.

There are increasing data available on the benefit of ACE inhibition in patients with diabetes from the point of view of both renal (see Chapter 3) and cardiovascular protection. In CAPPP [7], a subgroup of 572 patients with diabetes were allocated to receive either captopril or conventional therapy, to ascertain whether a diastolic blood pressure of less than 90 mmHg could be achieved. While there was no significant difference between conventional treatment and captopril treatment in patients without diabetes, in the subgroup with diabetes captopril treatment was associated with a significant reduction in myocardial infarction (34%) and all cardiac events (67%).

The recent HOPE study [6], which lasted 4.5 years, assessed the role of ACE inhibition in patients at high risk of cardiovascular events (see Chapter 4). A total of 9,297 high-risk patients, of whom 3,577 had diabetes, were included. The patients were at least 55 years old and the patients with diabetes had at least one other cardiovascular risk factor or a history of a previous cardiovascular event.

Patients were randomly allocated to receive placebo or ACE inhibition therapy (ramipril 10 mg/day). In the group with diabetes, ramipril treatment was associated with risk reduction of myocardial infarction (22%), stroke (33%), cardiovascular deaths (37%) and total mortality (24%) compared with placebo. Combined microvascular end points (overt nephropathy, dialysis or laser therapy for retinopathy) were significantly reduced (16%). Separate analysis of these end points did not, however, achieve statistical significance, but did show trends in favour of ACE inhibition therapy.

The CAPPP and HOPE studies have therefore confirmed the impressive benefit of ACE inhibition therapy in patients with diabetes, in terms of cardiovascular disease. With regard to microvascular disease, the EUCLID study [9] compared ACE inhibitor therapy (lisinopril) with placebo over two years [9], in a subgroup of 354 normotensive patients with type 1 diabetes and evaluable retinographs. The study showed evidence for renal protection (see Chapter 3) and a 45% reduction in the progression of retinopathy over the two-year follow-up period. The STENO II trial [10] reported similar findings, with a 45% reduction in the progression of retinopathy on an intensive treatment regimen, including ACE inhibition over a 3.8-year period. In contrast, the hypertension arm of the UKPDS showed no significant difference in the risk of microvascular complications when comparing atenolol treatment with captopril treatment in the group with tightly controlled blood pressure [11]. This led to the suggestion that it may be the blood pressure lowering per se, rather than ACE inhibition, that conferred particular benefit. This comparison within the UKPDS study was, however, not sufficiently powered to compare the different multiple antihypertensive regimens and the final answer is still awaited.

Table 5.2 summarizes the major clinically important conclusions from the most recent large, randomized, prospective trials, and these form a sound basis for a number of published guidelines for the management of hypertension associated with diabetes (see Chapter 6).

Questions not answered by the recent studies

A number of questions remain unanswered, particularly because not all classes of antihypertensive

Principal findings of the treatment trials of diabetes and hypertension
Type 2 diabetes hypertension treatment
• Reduces cardiovascular morbidity and mortality (evidence for thiazides, beta-blockers, ACE inhibitors and calcium antagonists)
• The threshold for intervention is $\geqslant$140/90 mmHg, with target of $\leqslant$140/80 mmHg
• More than 60% of patients will require two or more agents to achieve target blood pressure threshold
• Patient quality of life is not reduced and it is cost-effective
• Reduces progression of diabetic nephropathy
• Reduces progression of retinopathy and loss of visual acuity
Type 1 diabetes hypertension treatment
• Has not been shown to reduce cardiovascular end points
• Reduces progression of nephropathy in the incipient and overt phases
• The threshold for intervention is $\geqslant$140/90 mmHg, with target of <130/80 mmHg
• ACE inhibition has a specific renoprotective effect and may delay progression of retinopathy
• ACE inhibitors are recommended as first-line treatment

Table 5.2. ACE, angiotensin-converting enzyme.

drugs have been studied in randomized, controlled cardiovascular outcome studies. The usefulness of the newer antihypertensive agents such as angiotensin II antagonists in patients with diabetes are, as yet, unclear. These drugs appear to have good efficacy and good side-effect profiles, and are metabolically neutral. There is some evidence that patients with heart failure using angiotensin II antagonists will receive similar benefits to those using ACE inhibitors. Angiotensin II antagonists may also have a renoprotective effect. Alpha-blockers are also metabolically neutral, and may be of benefit in patients with diabetes. The role of alpha-blockers and angiotensin II antagonists is being elucidated by the ongoing Antihypertensive and Lipid Lowering Treatment to Prevent Heart Attack Trial (ALLHAT) [12]; however, following an interim analysis of the study, the alpha-blocker arm has been stopped prematurely, as this treatment was associated with a 1.25-fold increase in the relative risk of combined cardiovascular disease end points when compared with thiazide diuretic treatment. This difference was mainly related to an increase in the relative risk of heart failure and relative risk of stroke (1.19) [13].

Remaining issues include some controversy as to whether or not ACE inhibitors, particularly in type 2 diabetes, are superior to other agents in slowing the progression of diabetic nephropathy. There are also no randomized, controlled trials focusing on cardiovascular end points in type 1 diabetes.

More work needs to be performed in terms of diabetic retinopathy, particularly for elucidating whether or not ACE inhibitors have a specific effect on delaying presentation and progression of retinopathy over and above their blood pressure lowering effects [14]. In addition, angiotensin II antagonists have been suggested to have a similar role as ACE inhibitors and studies are planned to analyse this.

Finally, consideration of non-pharmacological therapy has not been included in recent treatment trials, although this remains an important adjunct to therapy. This is particularly relevant because of the multiple drug therapies commonly needed to achieve blood pressure targets and other targets such as glucose, glycated haemoglobin, and LDL-cholesterol, HDL-cholesterol and total cholesterol levels.

Summary

The principal findings of the recent hypertension controlled treatment trials in patients with diabetes confirmed the substantial benefit conferred in cardiovascular outcome, and showed that treatment of hypertension is cost-effective. The key values of blood pressure in patients with diabetes are a threshold of greater than 140/90 mmHg for intervention, with a target of less than 140/80 mmHg to be achieved on treatment. The safety and efficacy of ACE inhibitors, calcium antagonists, thiazide diuretics and beta-blocking agents has been confirmed. If the conclusions of the new studies are applied to all patients with diabetes, many more people with diabetes and hypertension will be alive and enjoying a better quality of life in the future.

References

1. Chowdhury TA, Kumar S, Barnett AH *et al.* **Treatment of hypertension in patients with type 2 diabetes: a review of the recent evidence.** *J Hum Hypertens* 1999, **13**: 803–811.

2. Curb JD, Pressel SL, Cutler *et al.* **Effect of diuretic-based antihypertensive treatment on cardiovascular disease risk in older diabetic patients with isolated systolic hypertension. Systolic Hypertension in the Elderly Program Cooperative Research Group.** *JAMA* 1996, **276**:1886–1892.

3. Anonymous. **Tight blood pressure control and risk of macrovascular complications in type 2 diabetes: UKPDS 38. UK Prospective Diabetes Study Group.** *Br Med J* 1998, **317**:703–713.

4. Hansson L, Zanchetti A, Carruthers SG *et al.* **Effects of intensive blood-pressure lowering and low-dose aspirin in patients with hypertension: principal results of the Hypertension Optimal Treatment (HOT) randomised trial. HOT Study Group.** *Lancet* 1998, **351**:1755–1762.

5. Tuomilehto J, Rastenyte D, Birkenhäger WH *et al.* **Effects of calcium-channel blockade in older subjects with diabetes and systolic hypertension. Systolic Hypertension in Europe Trial Investigators.** *N Engl J Med* 1999, **340**:677–684.

6. Anonymous. **Effects of ramipril on cardiovascular and microvascular outcomes in people with diabetes mellitus: results of the HOPE study and MICRO-HOPE substudy. Heart Outcomes Prevention Evaluation Study Investigators.** *Lancet* 2000, **355**:253–259.

7. Hansson L, Lindholm LH, Niskanen L *et al.* **Effect of angiotensin-converting-enzyme inhibition compared with conventional therapy on cardiovascular morbidity and mortality in hypertension: the Captopril Prevention Project (CAPPP) randomised trial.** *Lancet* 1999, **3543**:611–616.

8. Anonymous. **Cost effectiveness analysis of improved blood pressure control in hypertensive patients with type 2 diabetes: UKPDS 40. UK Prospective Diabetes Study Group.** *Br Med J* 1998, **317**:720–726.

9. Chaturvedi N, Sjolie AK, Stephenson JM *et al.* **Effect of lisinopril on progression of retinopathy in people with type 1 diabetes. The EUCLID Study Group. EURODIAB Controlled Trial of Lisinopril in Insulin-Dependent Diabetes Mellitus.** *Lancet* 1998, **351**:28–31.

10. Gaede P, Vedel P, Parving HH *et al.* **Intensified multifactorial intervention in patients with type 2 diabetes mellitus and microalbuminuria: the Steno type 2 randomised study.** *Lancet* 1999, **353**:617–622.

11. Anonymous. **Efficacy of atenolol and captopril in reducing risk of macrovascular and microvascular complications in type 2 diabetes: UKPDS 39. UK Prospective Diabetes Study Group.** *Br Med J* 1998, **317**:713–720.

12. Davis BR, Cutler JA, Gordon DJ *et al.* **Rationale and design for the Antihypertensive and Lipid Lowering Treatment to Prevent Heart Attack Trial (ALLHAT). ALLHAT Research Group.** *Am J Hypertens* 1996, **9**:342–360.

13. Beevers DG, Lip GYH. **Do alpha blockers cause heart failure and stroke? Observations from ALLHAT.** *J Hum Hypertens* 2000, **14**:287–289.

14. Gillow JT, Gibson JM, Dodson PM. **Hypertension and diabetic retinopathy – what's the story?** *Br J Ophthalmol* 1999, **83**:1083–1087.

Management of hypertension in the patient with diabetes

Until the 1980s, treatment of hypertension specifically in the patient with diabetes had not been the subject of detailed research. Recognition of hypertension as a significant factor for both macrovascular and microvascular disease [1,2] resulted in considerable interest as did the impressive data showing the delay in deterioration of renal function by treatment of hypertension. Diabetic patients with hypertension need separate consideration compared with their counterparts without diabetes for the following reasons:

- problems specifically associated with drug therapy (*see* Chapter 4);
- a high prevalence of other well-known cardiovascular risk factors (eg, hyperlipidaemia), which increases the risk for cardiovascular disease; and
- diabetic microvascular complications.

Although patients with type 1 and type 2 diabetes are considered separately, modern management puts particular emphasis on TOD (resulting from either macrovascular or microvascular disease). Recent data enforce the importance of management of hypertension in patients with incipient or overt diabetic nephropathy. The diabetic patient with hypertension poses special problems in diagnosis and clinical assessment.

Diagnosis

Hypertension was defined by the WHO and other national committees in 1999 as a diastolic blood pressure greater than 90 mmHg and/or systolic blood pressure greater than 140 mmHg [3]. A diagnosis of hypertension can be made when a number of separate readings confirm sustained, elevated blood pressure. Malignant or 'accelerated' hypertension is defined as hypertension associated with bilateral retinopathy including either exudation or haemorrhage [4,5], and may therefore be difficult to distinguish from diabetic retinopathy. Malignant hypertension may not be as rare as previously reported in the population with diabetes [4,6], as hypertensive retinal changes may be misclassified as diabetic retinopathy.

Care should be taken when measuring blood pressure, as obesity is common in the population with diabetes and it is important to use the correct sphygmomanometer cuff [7] (*see* Chapter 1). ABPM may be particularly valuable in patients with diabetes, helping to detect 'white coat' hypertension and guiding the estimation of blood pressure control with pharmacotherapy [8,9].

Clinical assessment and investigation

A number of important points must be considered during clinical assessment and investigation of the patient with diabetes and newly diagnosed hypertension (Tables 6.1–6.3). Emphasis should be placed on evidence of TOD (both macrovascular and microvascular disease), a search for other cardiovascular risk factors (to assess overall cardiovascular risk), contributory factors (eg, obesity, excess alcohol intake) and secondary causes. Simple investigations should be performed in all patients, including ECG, random serum cholesterol level and HDL-cholesterol level, as well as assessment of renal function and the presence of microalbuminuria and macroalbuminuria. The latter can be performed by using dipstick testing, 24-hour urine protein estimation or calculation of the urinary creatinine:albumin ratio. More specialized investigations (Table 6.4) should be considered if there is:

- resistant hypertension refractory to three or more agents;
- postural hypotension;
- suggestion of renal disease; and/or
- presence of accelerated hypertension.

Difficulties may arise in the diagnosis of accelerated hypertension in the patient with diabetes as the common retinal findings are found in both diabetes and hypertension (Figure 6.1). Indeed, accelerated hypertension may only be confirmed following effective antihypertensive treatment and close observation of resolution of retinal changes.

Clinical assessment of hypertension in the patient with diabetes

- Age and duration of diabetes
- Estimation of control of diabetes
- Therapy for diabetes (insulin or non-insulin)
- Family history of hypertension
- Family history of premature cardiovascular disease
- Smoker or non-smoker
- Alcohol intake
- Presence of complications of diabetes
- Drug history (eg, previous use of thiazide diuretics or steroids)
- History of hypertensive complications such as stroke, myocardial infarction or transient ischaemic attack
- Cardiovascular disease, including angina and intermittent claudication
- Previous urinary tract infection or renal disease
- History appropriate to secondary causes of hypertension associated with diabetes

Table 6.1

Clinical examination of hypertension in the patient with diabetes

- Degree and type of hypertension (eg, isolated diastolic, systolic or combined form)
- Correction for obesity with measurement of blood pressure
- Presence of clinical signs of hypertension, such as displaced apex beat and left ventricular hypertrophy
- Complications of diabetes (eg, retinopathy [hypertensive or diabetic], carotid stenosis, coronary heart disease and peripheral vascular disease)
- Signs of associated hyperlipidaemia
- Signs of coexisting renal disease (renal artery bruits)
- Signs associated with other endocrinopathies and secondary causes

Table 6.2

Investigation of hypertension in the patient with diabetes

- Chest radiography for cardiomegaly
- ECG, to establish ischaemic heart disease or left ventricular hypertrophy, and left anterior hemiblock
- Urea, creatinine and electrolytes to establish presence of established renal disease
- Urine, for proteinuria (incipient or established diabetic nephropathy), and culture and sensitivity, for signs of urinary tract infection
- Random serum cholesterol and triglyceride estimation, to establish concomitant hyperlipidaemia, especially hypercholesterolaemia
- Glycosylated haemoglobin or fructosamine, for level of control of diabetes
- Other endocrine tests may be appropriate, for example:
  - 24-hour urinary catecholamines estimation for phaeochromocytoma
  - Random growth hormone or insulin growth factor 1 for acromegaly
  - Free thyroxine and thyroxine stimulating hormone for thyrotoxicosis

Table 6.3. ECG, electrocardiograph.

Specialized investigations for assessing diabetic patients with hypertension

- Ultrasound of kidneys
- Renal arteriography
- Renal biopsy
- Urinary catecholamine estimation
- Autonomic nerve function tests

Table 6.4

The role of renal biopsy in diabetic patients with hypertension and elevated serum creatinine should be mentioned. The majority of these patients have underlying nephrosclerosis and manifest changes of diabetic nephropathy [10]. Other types of renal disease have been identified, for example, glomerulonephritis of the membranous type and pyelonephritis. The decision to perform a renal biopsy depends on the duration of diabetes, the evolution of the nephropathy and the presence of other microangiopathic complications; for example, a renal biopsy may be justified in a patient with type 1 diabetes with proteinuria and diabetes of less than eight years' duration, or in the absence of retinopathy.

Renal artery stenosis poses a special problem. It is likely from the limited prevalence data available (*see* Chapter 1) that the condition is more common in patients with diabetes, but may not be haemodynamically significant in many cases [12]. In clinical practice, marked deterioration in renal function with ACE inhibitor therapy is, fortunately, rare.

Diabetic neuropathic ulcer

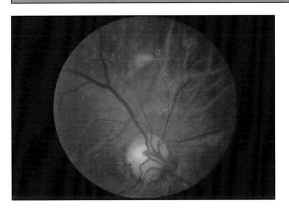
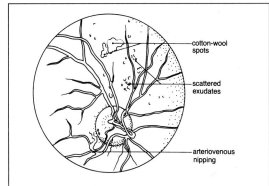
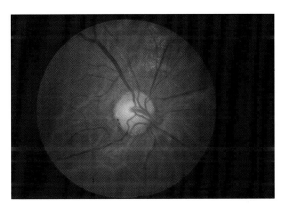
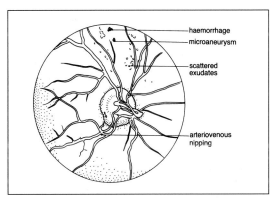

Figure 6.1. The retinographs are of the left retina of a West Indian woman with diabetes and severe hypertension. Do they show predominantly diabetic or hypertensive retinopathy? The abnormalities include cotton-wool spots (a), microaneurysms (b) and haemorrhage, widespread exudation and arteriovenous nipping (a and b). While these appearances were originally thought to be caused by accelerated hypertension rather than diabetes, antihypertensive treatment subsequently diminished the retinal abnormalities and macular exudation, probably owing to the diabetes, developed.

Management of hypertension in patients with diabetes

Previously, the management of hypertension associated with diabetes was based on extrapolation of data from large treatment trials in patients without diabetes in conjunction with the clear benefits of lowering blood pressure on the progression of diabetic nephropathy. A large evidence base concerning antihypertensive treatment in patients with diabetes is now available that has clarified the exact benefit, the goals of therapy and the safety of many of the classes of blood pressure drugs available (*see* Chapter 5 and Table 5.1). Guidelines for management have, therefore, been updated [3,12–14].

Once the diagnosis of hypertension is established, a decision needs to be made on whether pharmacological treatment be instituted as first-line therapy, in addition to general lifestyle measures. Table 6.5 shows the clinical situations requiring initial drug therapy, with emphasis on secondary prevention (ie, presence of clinical evidence of macrovascular disease), TOD and degree of overall cardiovascular risk of the individual.

Patients with diabetes and established hypertension should be screened for secondary causes, particularly the regular use of drugs with pressor potential (eg, alcohol, oral contraceptives, non-steroidal anti-inflammatory agents, liquorice and steroids). If clinical or routine laboratory features suggest a secondary cause, investigations should be performed to exclude thyroid dysfunction, phaeochromocytoma, Cushing's syndrome, Conn's syndrome, acromegaly, and renal artery stenosis.

The importance of overall cardiovascular risk assessment in guiding the therapeutic decisions is discussed below.

Cardiovascular risk assessment

Patients with CHD are at high absolute risk of a further vascular event over subsequent years. This group of patients is, therefore, considered for secondary prevention, and cardiovascular risk assessment is unnecessary. Targets and thresholds for treatment in this context are well-established. Individuals without CHD may, however, still be at greater risk for it when compared with the healthy population, as a result of the coexistent and additive effects of multiple risk factors, such as patients with diabetes.

Assessment of absolute CHD risk takes into account the influence of major CHD risk factors for an individual and their annual expression as five-year or 10-year risk. Study of epidemiological and prospective follow-up data from, for example, the Multiple Risk Factor Intervention Trial (MRFIT), Prospective Cardiovascular Münster Study (PRO-CAM) and Framingham studies, has allowed such a calculation for an individual [14–17]. The most widely used and validated equation is based on the Framingham study and may now be calculated on sophisticated computerized programs [17]. This equation has been used as the basis of cardiovascular risk assessment in the guidelines of the WHO, joint British societies', BHS and JNC-VI (USA) [3,12–14]. An example of these calculations is shown in Figure 6.2 [18], which shows the data required, with a resultant 10-year CHD risk calculated for an individual.

Clinical indications for pharmacological treatment of hypertension in patients with diabetes
• Patients with evidence of incipient or established nephropathy
• Pregnant
• Accelerated or severe hypertension
• Blood pressure >140/90 mmHg and: - Evidence of macrovascular disease and/or   - Left ventricular hypertrophy and/or   - Diabetic retinopathy
• Blood pressure >140/90 mmHg with: - Cardiovascular risk: >15% 10 year CHD risk and   - No evidence of vascular disease or target organ damage and   - No response to target levels with lifestyle measures

Table 6.5. CHD, chronic heart disease.

Assessment of cardiovascular risk

Form

Coronary heart disease risk request

Does NOT apply to patients with ischaemic heart disease, peripheral vascular disease or genetic hyperlipidaemia

Age:	....	(30–74 years only)
Sex:	M .... F	
Systolic blood pressure:	.... mmHg	(mean of last two readings)
Cigarette smoker:	Yes .... No	(no = not for at least 12 months)
Paitent with diabetes:	Yes .... No	
ECG shows LVH:	Yes .... No .... Don't know	

Example

Coronary heart disease risk analysis

Age:	66 years
Sex:	Male
Systolic blood pressure:	170 mmHg
Cigarette smoker:	No
Patient with diabetes:	Yes
ECG shows LVH:	No
Blood tests:	Total cholesterol = 5.3 mmol/l (3.6–6.5)
	HDL-cholesterol = 1.00 mmol/l (0.60–1.60)
Result:	10-year coronary heart disease risk = 31.3%

Risk calculated using the Framingham equation

Calculation valid for those subjects aged 30–74 years only

Does not apply to those with ischaemic heart disease or genetic hyperlipidaemia

Figure 6.2. The assessment was calculated from the Framingham equation information required from the clinician (a) and an example of coronary risk analysis (b). M, male; F, female; LVH, left ventricular hypertrophy; ECG, electrocardiograph; HDL, high-density lipoprotein. Reproduced with permission from [18].

Note that the data entry includes only well-known risk factors and, in particular, does not include:

- ethnic origin (eg, Asians are at higher risk);
- presence of proteinuria (increased risk);
- family history of premature coronary heart disease;
- patients younger than 30 years or older than 74 years of age; and
- risk conferred by genetic hyperlipidaemia.

This system is simple and robust but it does not include diastolic blood pressure or serum triglyceride levels, the latter negating the need for fasting blood samples. Calculations of the degree of lowering risk, by risk factor intervention (including target levels), are easily made, with the potential for patient education.

The exact lower threshold level of cardiovascular risk that requires intervention, particularly pharmacological intervention, is still contentious. In situations where resources are limited, it is imperative to direct drug treatment to individuals of high or very high risk (ie, greater than 30% risk of an event over 10 years or greater than 3% risk of an event over one year): this was the initial advice of the Standing Medical Advisory Committee (SMAC) in the UK. Subsequent guidelines have lowered this threshold to greater than 15% risk of CHD over 10 years (joint British societies', BHS and WHO recommendations) [3,13,14]. The lower threshold will have a considerable impact on clinical practice in terms of manpower, patient compliance, multiple drug therapies and resource allocation in patients with diabetes. For example, a recent study of cardiovascular risk in 1,060 patients with diabetes attending a hospital clinic for an annual review of diabetes demonstrated that 43% of patients had a risk of greater than 20% 10-year CHD risk (>2% per year) and 20% greater than 30% 10-year CHD risk (>3% per year) [17]. The authors' suggest that greater than 20% 10-year CHD risk is a more realistic current lower threshold, but the aim in the longer term is for this threshold to be 15% 10-year CHD absolute risk.

Thresholds and goals of therapy based on the clinical trials

Antihypertensive therapy is indicated in patients with diabetes if the threshold of systolic blood pressure (140 mmHg or greater) or diastolic blood pressure (90 mmHg or greater) is consistently breached [3]. Table 6.5 demonstrates the concept that low cardiovascular risk in an individual allows a trial of only non-pharmacological therapy.

The recent large treatment trials (*see* Chapter 5) have clarified the use of suggested target blood pressure during antihypertensive treatment with both systolic and diastolic blood pressure targets being achieved together; these targets are shown in Table 6.6 [13]. Even lower targets of blood pressure should be aimed for in patients with type 1 diabetes who have 1 g or greater proteinuria per 24-hour urine collection. The low blood pressure targets for both type 1 and type 2 diabetes are indeed a challenge to patients and their carers.

Choice of pharmacological therapy

The recent trials have provided evidence for the benefit of treatment of hypertension in patients with diabetes, particularly type 2 patients (*see*

Chapter 5) [19]. This has made rational prescribing choices more straightforward, although a number of questions have not, as yet, been answered [19]. The early trials of antihypertensive therapy commonly used thiazide diuretics and beta-blocking agents, but these were thought to be disadvantageous in patients with diabetes because of the increased risk of deterioration in other metabolic factors (eg, glycaemic control and hypertriglyceridaemia). In contrast, new evidence has shown that low dose thiazide, beta-blocker, calcium antagonist and ACE inhibitor drug groups are safe and effective with respect to cardiovascular outcome. In addition, the renoprotective effect of ACE inhibitors is well established in type 1 diabetes [20,21] and data is accumulating that suggests this is also true in type 2 diabetes [20–22].

Although evidence for the effects of the newer antihypertensive agents on long-term outcome is, as yet, not available, angiotensin II antagonists, specific alpha-blockers and centrally acting drugs (eg, moxonidine) are metabolically neutral, lower blood pressure and are well-tolerated. These groups of agents, therefore, currently constitute second-line therapy, with the angiotensin II antagonists being an appropriate choice if an ACE inhibitor cannot be tolerated, usually because of persistent cough. Contraindications and specific indications for the different classes of antihypertensive agents have been outlined in Chapter 4.

The impressive and consistent data on the renal and cardiovascular protection affected by ACE inhibitors, position this group of drugs as the preferred first-line therapy. Calcium antagonists, beta-blockers, and thiazides are suitable first-line alternatives in patients with type 1 or type 2 diabetes. In the management plan (Figure 6.3), it must be emphasised that the majority of diabetic patients with hypertension will require at least two antihypertensive drugs

Target blood pressures during antihypertensive treatment		
	Clinic blood pressure	ABPM or home blood pressure
Optimal blood pressure	<140/80 mmHg	<130/75 mmHg
Audit standard	<140/85 mmHg	<140/80 mmHg

Table 6.6. ABPM, ambulatory blood pressure day time means; home blood pressure, measured with validated automated electronic devices. Reproduced with permission from [13].

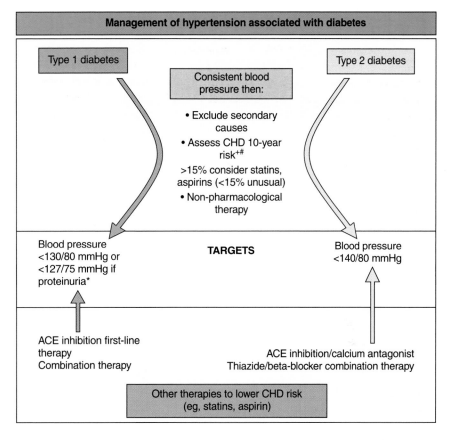

Figure 6.3. +, coronary heart disease risk calculated by Framingham equation; #, in the context of secondary prevention (ie, existing coronary heart disease) statins (or fibrates) and aspirin are appropriate; *proteinuria >1 g/day; CHD, chronic heart disease; ACE, angiotensin-converting enzyme. Serum cholesterol target <4.8 mmol/l.

to achieve tight blood pressure targets, such that combination therapy will become standard practice; other therapies (eg, statins and aspirin) are an integral part of management. Further guidance will be provided by the presence of pre-existing cardiovascular disease and a 10-year CHD risk analysis using the Framingham equation.

The role of non-pharmacological therapy in the treatment of diabetes has long been established and in clinical practice dietary measures, cessation of smoking and of intake of excess alcohol, encouraging exercise, and reduction of stress, all have a role in the therapeutic management of diabetes (Table 6.7). Studies have shown that the principles of dietary intake advised for patients with diabetes (increasing unrefined carbohydrate and fibre intake and lowering fat to 30% of total energy intake per day), has significant blood pressure lowering effects (eg, systolic and diastolic blood pressure −17 mmHg and −10 mmHg, respectively, over one year) [23]. Moderate sodium restriction or weight loss alone, are sufficient to produce clinically significant

blood pressure reductions [24]. These interventions alone or in combination may reduce the need for drug therapy and enhance the effects of antihypertensive agents, but their favourable effects on outcome are only assumed, and not proven.

Principal non-pharmacological measures for therapeutic management of diabetes
Reduction: • weight • salt intake • fat intake • saturated fat intake • alcohol intake (<2 units/day) • smoking (cessation, if possible) **Increase:** • fibre intake • unrefined carbohydrate • polyunsaturated and monosaturated fats • exercise

Table 6.7

Type 1 diabetic patients with hypertension

Initial management in type 1 diabetic patients with hypertension should include clinical assessment and investigation. Most of these patients have essential hypertension, and management for them is as suggested in Figure 6.3. Emphasis should be placed on the presence of TOD, particularly the presence of nephropathy, which is usually underlying. Blood pressure lowering, particularly with ACE inhibitor treatment, slows the decline of renal function in overt nephropathy and delays progression from the microalbuminuria phase, such that ACE inhibitors are recommended as first-line therapy [13,21,22,24]. To achieve renoprotection, tight blood pressure control is of upmost importance and combinations of antihypertensive drugs are usually required. Thiazides, calcium antagonists and cardioselective beta-blockers and alpha-blockers are all suitable (avoiding class contra-indications) [13].

The use of ACE inhibitors may also be indicated in the presence of diabetic retinopathy. The EUCLID (patients with type 1 diabetes) and HOPE (patients with type 2 diabetes) studies have demonstrated encouraging results for both lisinopril and ramipril in delaying progression of retinopathy (EUCLID 48% reduction in progression, HOPE trend to reduction in laser therapy) [25,26].

The thresholds and targets of blood pressure for diagnosis and treatment are shown in Table 6.6 and Figure 6.3. Possible therapeutic combinations include an ACE inhibitor with a diuretic (loop or thiazide), ACE inhibitor and calcium antagonist, or a combination including an alpha-blocker. Angiotensin II antagonists are effective alone or in combination, and are particularly indicated when cough is a clinical problem caused by ACE inhibitors. Caution is required with any ACE inhibitor/diuretic combination to avoid the first-dose effect of a sudden large drop in blood pressure. To avoid this, diuretics should be stopped for several days before instituting treatment with an ACE inhibitor. Renal function should be checked one week after starting ACE inhibitor treatment, as those rare patients with previously unknown renal artery stenosis can experience rapid deterioration in renal function.

Patients with type 1 diabetes who show evidence of nephropathy are at a very high risk of cardiovascular disease. Therefore, they may be considered for statin therapy and aspirin. Patients with type 1 diabetes and no evidence of diabetic nephropathy or pre-existing cardiovascular disease should have management guided by CHD risk assessment (ie, above or below 15% 10-year CHD threshold, suggested by the joint British societies' guidelines) [14].

Special mention should be made of the patient with type 1 diabetes and persistent microalbuminuria or proteinuria and normotension (see Chapter 3). Evidence is accumulating that these patients may benefit from ACE inhibitor therapy, but it remains unclear whether this benefit is derived from associated blood pressure reduction or a specific ACE inhibition effect.

Type 2 diabetic patients with hypertension

Hypertension in the population with type 2 diabetes has a high prevalence, estimated at greater than 60% with the current diagnostic blood pressure criteria (blood pressure of 140/90 mmHg or greater). It is strongly related to obesity, hyperlipidaemia, low HDL-cholesterol, and is highly predictive of cardiovascular and microvascular complications. The UKPDS has also demonstrated that many patients with type 2 diabetes (approximately 50%) have evidence of established cardiovascular or microvascular disease at diagnosis [1]. In addition, 40% of patients with type 2 diabetes have a 10-year CHD risk of greater than 20% (>2% per year). Initial clinical assessment should therefore focus not just on hypertension and its aetiology, but on the presence of TOD and overall cardiovascular risk.

Initial therapy should address non-pharmacological therapy, assessing potential for weight reduction, cessation of smoking, encouraging exercise and dietary manipulation (Table 6.7). In most instances, however, this will not be sufficient to lower blood pressure to the tight targets now established (Table 6.6 and Figure 6.3), such that pharmacological therapy, often two or more antihypertenisve drugs, will be required [27,28].

The choice of drug therapy for hypertension in patients with type 2 diabetes is less clear cut. Four classes of antihypertensive drugs (ACE inhibitor, calcium antagonist, thiazide diuretic and beta-blocker) have been shown to be beneficial for cardiovascular and microvascular outcomes. The case for ACE inhibition as the preferred first-line therapy has been supported by the HOPE and CAPPP studies [26,29], while the comparison of beta-blocker therapy with ACE inhibition therapy in the hypertension arm of the UKPDS [30] demonstrated no difference. The ongoing ALLHAT and other trials, which include comparative studies of alpha-blockers and angiotensin II antagonists, may determine which agent should be chosen as the first-line treatment. The presence of TOD may, however, provide guidance on initial drug choice. For example, angina is common in patients with type 2 diabetes and initial appropriate therapy would be a beta-blocker or calcium antagonist, whereas the presence of peripheral vascular disease contraindicates beta-blockers. Like patients with type 1 diabetes and hypertension, combination therapies are likely to be required to achieve blood pressure targets.

In the presence of diabetic nephropathy, there is less evidence to guide clinical practice in patients with type 2 diabetes, as compared with patients with type 1 diabetes. Although blood pressure reduction is vital, it is less clear whether ACE inhibition *per se* has a specific renoprotective action beyond blood pressure reduction [20–22]. This conclusion is similar with regard to diabetic retinopathy [31].

The high cardiovascular risk of patients with type 2 diabetes suggests that a more 'holistic' approach to management should be adopted, with therapeutic strategies other than blood pressure and glycaemic control being offered. Aspirin should be offered to all type 2 diabetic patients with hypertension, providing there is good blood pressure control and no contraindications (eg, allergy, potential site for haemorrhage). Many patients will require statin therapy for primary prevention because their estimated 10-year CHD risk is 15% or greater.

Summary

Hypertension (blood pressure, $\geqslant 140/90$ mmHg) is common in people with diabetes. Data in diabetic patients with hypertension have shown proven benefit in reduction of cardiovascular disease with antihypertensive therapy. In addition, there is clear evidence that antihypertensive therapy in the presence of diabetic nephropathy slows decline in renal function and may reduce the progression of retinopathy in patients with type 1 diabetes.

Management should include overall cardiovascular risk assessment and investigation to find a primary or secondary cause. While non-pharmacological advice is appropriate for all patients with diabetes and hypertension, two or more antihypertensive drugs are likely to be required to achieve tight blood pressure in the majority.

ACE inhibitors are the preferred first-line therapy in patients with type 1 and type 2 diabetes, although in patients with type 2 diabetes, calcium antagonists, thiazides and cardioselective beta-blockers have proven benefit and safety. Blood pressure lowering to the recommended target levels is of paramount importance. Available evidence should encourage all clinicians caring for patients with diabetes to make a significant impact on cardiovascular mortality that is cost-effective and should include a more holistic approach to treatment of overall cardiovascular risk, including lipid-lowering agents and aspirin.

References

1. Staessen JA, Thijs L, Fagard R *et al*. **Predicting cardiovascular risk using conventional vs ambulatory blood pressure in older patients with systolic hypertension. Systolic Hypertension in Europe Trial Investigators.** *JAMA* 1999, **282**:539–546.

2. Parving HH, Hommel E. **Prognosis in diabetic nephropathy.** *Br Med J* 1989, **299**:230–233.

3. Anonymous. **1999 World Health Organisation-International Society of Hypertension Guidelines for the Management of Hypertension. Guidelines Subcommittee.** *J Hypertens* 1999, **17**:151–183.

4. Dodson PM, Lip GYH, Eames SM *et al*. **Hypertensive retinopathy: a review of existing classification systems and a suggestion for a simplified grading system.** *J Hum Hypertens* 1996, **10**:93–98.

5. McGregor E, Isles CG, Jay JL *et al*. **Retinal changes in malignant hypertension.** *Br Med J* 1986, **292**:233–234.

6. Drury PL. **Diabetes and arterial hypertension.** *Diabetologia* 1983, **24**:1–9.

7. Weidmann P, Boehlen LM, de Courten M *et al*. **Antihypertensive therapy in diabetic patients.** *J Hum Hypertens* 1992, **6** (suppl. 2):S23–S36.

8. Kaplan NM. **Ambulatory blood pressure monitoring: valuable in diabetic subjects?** *Diab Rev Int* 1996, **5**:11–14.

9. Stergiou GS, Skeva II, Zoubaki AS *et al*. **Self-monitoring of blood pressure at home: how many measurements are needed?** *J Hypertens* 1998, **16**:725–731.

10. Ditscherlein G. **Renal histopathology in hypertensive diabetic patients.** *Hypertension* 1985, **7**:II29–32.

11. Eardley KS, Lipkin GW. **Atherosclerotic renal artery stenosis: is it worth diagnosing?** *J Hum Hypertens* 1999, **13**:271–220.

12. Anonymous. **The sixth report of the Joint National Committee on prevention, detection, evaluation, and**

treatment of high blood pressure. *Arch Intern Med* 1997, **157**:2413–2446.

13. Ramsay L, Williams B, Johnston G *et al.* **Guidelines for management of hypertension: report of the third working party of the British Hypertension Society.** *J Hum Hypertens* 1999, **13**:569–592.

14. Anonymous. **Joint British recommendations on prevention of coronary heart disease in clinical practice. British Cardiac Society, British Hyperlipidaemia Association, British Hypertension Society, endorsed by the British Diabetic Association.** *Heart* 1998, **80** (suppl. 2):S1–S29.

15. Wilson PW, D'Agostino RB, Levy D *et al.* **Prediction of coronary heart disease using risk factor categories.** *Circulation* 1998, **97**:1837–1847.

16. Kannel WB. **Fifty years of Framingham study contributions to understanding hypertension.** *J Hum Hypertens* 2000, **14**:83–90.

17. Bayly GR, Barlett WA, Davies PH *et al.* **Laboratory-based calculation of coronary heart disease risk in a hospital diabetic clinic.** *Diabet Med* 1999, **16**:697–701.

18. PM Dodson, AH Barnett. *Lipids in Primary Care.* London: Medical Publishing Company, 1999;45.

19. Chowdhury TA, Kumar S, Barnett AH *et al.* **Treatment of hypertension in patients with type 2 diabetes: a review of the recent evidence.** *J Hum Hypertens* 1999, **13**:803–811.

20. Cooper ME. **Pathogenesis, prevention, and treatment of diabetic nephropathy.** *Lancet* 1998, **352**:213–219.

21. Mogensen CE, Keane WF, Bennett PH *et al.* **Prevention of diabetic renal disease with special reference to microalbuminuria.** *Lancet* 1995, **346**:1080–1084.

22. Parving HH. **Initiation and progression of diabetic nephropathy.** *N Engl J Med* 1996, **335**:1682–1683.

23. Dodson PM, Pacy PJ, Bal P *et al.* **A controlled trial of a high fibre, low fat and low sodium diet for mild hypertension in type 2 (non-insulin-dependent) diabetic patients.** *Diabetologia* 1984, **27**:522–526.

24. Dodson PM, Beevers M, Hallworth R *et al.* **Sodium restriction and blood pressure in hypertensive type II diabetics: randomised blind controlled and crossover studies of moderate sodium restriction and sodium supplementation.** *Br Med J* 1989, **298**:227–230.

25. Chaturvedi N, Sjolie AU, Stephenson JM *et al.* **Effect of lisinopril on progression of retinopathy in people with type 1 diabetes. The EUCLID Study Group. EURODIAB Controlled Trial of Lisinopril in Insulin-Dependent Diabetes Mellitus.** *Lancet* 1998, **351**:28–31.

26. Anonymous. **Effects of ramipril on cardiovascular and microvascular outcomes in people with diabetes mellitus: results of the HOPE study and MICRO-HOPE substudy. Heart Outcomes Prevention Evaluation Study Investigators.** *Lancet* 2000, **355**:253–259.

27. Hansson L, Zanchetti A, Carruthers SG *et al.* **Effects of intensive blood-pressure lowering and low-dose aspirin in patients with hypertension: principal results of the Hypertension Optimal Treatment (HOT) randomised trial. HOT Study Group.** *Lancet* 1998, **351**:1755–1762.

28. Anonymous. **Tight blood pressure control and risk of macrovascular complications in type 2 diabetes: UKPDS 38. UK Prospective Diabetes Study Group.** *Br Med J* 1998, **317**:703–713.

29. Hansson L, Lindholm LH, Niskanen L *et al.* **Effect of angiotensin-converting-enzyme inhibition compared with conventional therapy on cardiovascular morbidity and mortality in hypetension: the Captopril Prevention Project (CAPPP) randomised trial.** *Lancet* 1999, **353**:611–616.

30. Anonymous. **Efficacy of atenolol and captopril in reducing risk of macrovascular and microvascular complications in type 2 diabetes: UKPDS 39. UK Prospective Diabetes Study Group.** *Br Med J* 1998, **317**:713–720.

31. Gillow JT, Gibson JM, Dodson PM. **Hypertension and diabetic retinopathy – what's the story?** *Br J Ophthalmol* 1999, **83**:1083–1087.

Index